DON'T COUNT YOURSELF OUT

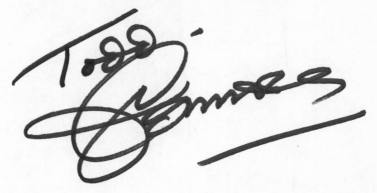

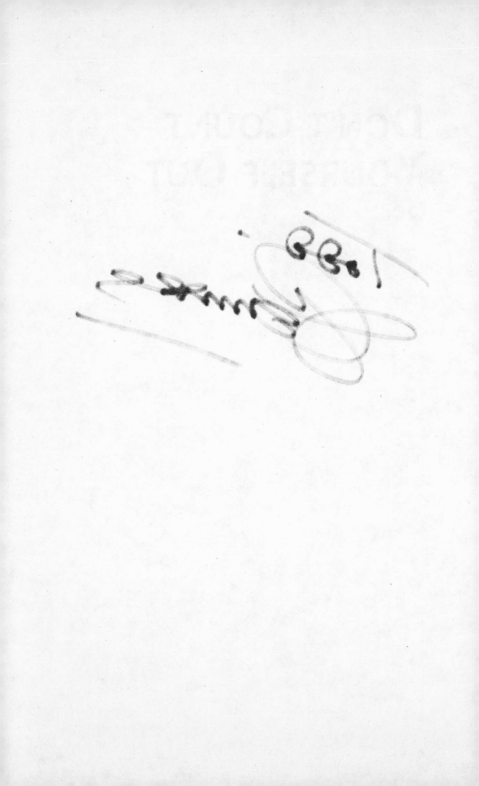

DON'T
COUNT
YOURSELF
OUT

STAYING FIT AFTER 35

JIMMY CONNORS
with NEIL GORDON, M.D., Ph.D.,
and Catherine McEvily Harris

HYPERION

New York

Figure 3-1 reprinted by permission of Simon & Schuster. Copyright © 1991, Rosenberg, Evans, and Thompson; Figure 3-2 adapted from *Journal of the American Medical Association* 1990; 263: 3029–3034, Copyright © 1990, American Medical Association; Figure 3-4 adapted from *Journal of the American Medical Association* 1989; 262: 2395–2401, Copyright © 1989, American Medical Association; Figure 4-1 adapted from *American Journal of Cardiology* 1990; 65: 1010–1013. Copyright © 1990, American Journal of Cardiology; Figures 4-2 and 4-3 adapted from *Journal of the American Medical Association* 1991; 266: 3295–3299, Copyright © 1991, American Medical Association; Figure 4-4 adapted from *Medicine and Science in Sports and Exercise* 1982; 114: 377–387, Copyright © 1982, The American College of Sports Medicine. The CONNORS COUNT health and fitness points system is a trademark of Jimmy Connors and Neil Gordon, M.D., Ph.D.

Library of Congress Cataloging-in-Publication Data
Connors, Jimmy, 1952-
     Don't count yourself out : staying fit after 35 with Jimmy
  Connors / by Jimmy Connors with Neil Gordon and Catherine
McEvily Harris.—1st ed.
     p. cm.
  ISBN 1-56282-927-0 : $22.95
  1. Physical fitness. 2. Exercise. I. Gordon, Neil F.
II. Harris, Catherine McEvily. III. Title.
GV481.C654 1992
796.7'044—dc20   92-18464
                                                        CIP

First Edition
10 9 8 7 6 5 4 3 2 1

This book is dedicated to

MY MOM, GLORIA, AND TO MY GRANDMOTHER,
TWO-MOM,
two women who taught me a man's game
and who never let me forget from where I came.

TO MY WIFE PATTI, MY SON BRETT,
AND MY DAUGHTER, AUBREE,
whose understanding, patience, and love
enabled me to continue the grind.

TO ALL THE GREAT FANS
I HAVE MET OVER THE YEARS.
Thank you for being part of my career.

To my wife, Tracey,
and daughters, Kim and Terri,
for being more than any man
could ever wish for.
Neil Gordon, M.D., Ph.D.

Contents

Acknowledgments   ix
Introduction   Forty Love   1

PART ONE   COUNTING YOURSELF IN

Chapter 1   Don't Count Me Out   11
Chapter 2   Being Fit. What Does It Mean?   26
Chapter 3   What's in It for You?   32
Chapter 4   The Million-Dollar Question: How
Much Is Enough?   50
Chapter 5   Don't Work Your Lifestyle—Make
Your Lifestyle Work   75

PART TWO   THE JIMMY CONNORS WORKOUT PROGRAM—

FEATURING THE CONNORS COUNT

Chapter 6   Practicing Safe Exercise   91
Chapter 7   16 Weeks to a Lifetime of Fitness   107

PART THREE   FIT FOR THE FUTURE

Chapter 8   Eliminating the F Word   217
Chapter 9   Beyond Exercise   228

Afterword The Ball's in Your Court 237

Selected Bibliography 239

Index 241

Acknowledgments

WORKING TOGETHER ON THIS BOOK has been an extremely enjoyable and gratifying experience. To provide you, the reader, with the best we have to offer, we have required the assistance and cooperation of many talented people. While they are too numerous to list, we would like to recognize a few special contributions.

Catherine McEvily Harris, an exceptionally gifted writer based in Los Angeles, California, successfully blended our personal thoughts and medical knowledge into words that everyone can understand and enjoy. Cathy's recommendations and overall contributions to the book were invaluable.

Our editor at Hyperion, Judith Riven, not only provided guidance that greatly enhanced the practical value of the book but was a pleasure to work with.

Herb Katz, Ed Brennan, and Ray Benton were extremely helpful in expediting the business arrangements for the book. Herb and his partner, Nancy Katz, our literary agents, also provided valuable editorial assistance.

Dr. Joel Woodburn, our mutual friend, was responsible for bringing us together and was a big help every step of the way. Joel and Bill Lelly, Jimmy's lifelong friend and assistant, were responsible for coordinating schedules so that the book could get completed in a timely fashion.

Gloria Connors provided lengthy interviews for the book and helped in many other ways. Patti, Brett, and Aubree Connors graciously shared the limited time they have with Jimmy so that we could get this book done right.

Sheila Burford and Laura Becker helped with the typing of the manuscript and compilation of the figures and charts. Dean Stevenson, a Phoenix, Arizona, photographer took the photos of Jimmy doing the various stretching and muscle-strengthening exercises.

Chris Scott, M.S., John Duncan, Ph.D., Randy Kennedy, B.E.S., and many of Neil's colleagues at the Cooper Institute for Aerobics Research, Dallas, Texas, provided much after-hours scientific guidance, feedback, and support.

To all these people, and the many others we have not listed, much thanks!

Jimmy Connors
Neil Gordon, M.D., Ph.D.

Introduction: Forty Love

"We may be witnessing Jimmy Connors' final trip to this tournament. Although there's been no talk of retirement yet, this great champion is now considered an old man in tennis."

THAT QUOTE was taken from a sports commentator during the 1982 U.S. Open. I was 30 years old. I wonder what that guy must have thought when I made it to the semifinals at the U.S. Open after celebrating my 39th birthday in 1991 and what he thinks about the fact that I'm *still* competing now at age 40. Chances are, *he's* the one who has retired.

I've been called the ageless wonder of tennis, the ol' man river of tennis, the father of tennis, and the grandfather of tennis! Where is it written that 40 is *old?* And even if it is written somewhere, who says it's true? I may be 40, but I don't know when, if ever, I've felt more alive or more in control of my life than I do today. I don't believe I have to quit playing tennis or anything else just because I'm 40.

Yet I'm continually asked when I'm going to hang up the racquet. Quite frankly, I'm a little tired of being asked when I'm going to quit. I'll stop playing professional tennis when I can no longer contribute to the quality of the sport or when the sport is no longer contributing to the quality of my life. I'll know when. I'll feel it in my gut. It's for me to decide—no one else. Those who count me out before my time will continue to be surprised. Those who have counted me out before my time are part of the reason I'm still around. Motivation comes from a lot of different places.

Rather than ask when I'll retire, the more important question, I think, is how have I lasted longer in my profession than most of my peers? It hasn't been by accident, I assure you. And it's not a mystery, at least not to me. Through years of experience I've discovered precisely how much exercise I need to stay in peak physical condition. That's the secret to my success—knowing how much exercise my own body needs. Too much and I'd get burned out. Too little and I wouldn't be able to compete with the young guys.

The key to knowing how much exercise I need is so simple that it's easy to overlook. When my body talks to me, I listen. Like everyone else's, my body is constantly sending me important messages. These messages tell me things like when to eat, when to stop eating, when I need water, and when I need sleep. But my body also tells me other things, things most people haven't learned to interpret. It tells me when I'm overdoing my training, when I'm being too easy on myself, when I can afford to skip a workout, and when it's time to push harder. By carefully tuning in to my body, an ability instilled in me a long time ago by my mom and grandmother, I have been able to stay at the top of a physically demanding sport for a lot of years.

When I was first approached about writing a book on this fitness regime, I was hesitant—particularly when it was suggested that the book be targeted to men and women over 35 who are not interested in being competitive athletes. I don't like it when people tell me what to do and I was uncomfortable with the idea of dictating to others—especially to the fans who have been so loyal to me. I also know that most people have neither the intent nor the desire to follow an exercise program designed to meet the needs of a professional tennis player. Why should they? Hell, if I weren't competing, I'd do what I had to do to look good and be healthy—period. Today I may exercise so that I can last five hours on the court with kids half my age, but ten years from now I'll be exercising for other reasons altogether—to prevent a heart attack, to keep up with my children, and to fit into the jeans I'm wearing right now. The demand for the intensity at which I work out today will no longer be there. But I'll still have the need to exercise because I want to stay active. We all exercise for different reasons at different times of our lives.

But then it occurred to me that my exercise program could be modified so that men and women at any level of fitness would benefit. I could teach people to understand the language of the body. If I developed the method I use into a system that would be easy to follow, anyone would be able to figure out the amount of exercise they need regardless of their physical goals. Some may want to look better, others may want to feel better. Some people exercise to release stress, others exercise to become fitter and healthier. Knowing the amount of exercise needed to achieve any or all of these goals would make the concept of exercise so much easier. What better way of giving something back to those who have stuck it out with me for all these years?

I knew my workout could be adapted to fit many needs because nothing I do is all that complicated. I travel a great deal, so I don't always have access to a gym. I have to improvise. When I'm not on the road, my first priority is my family. I need a workout that can fit into my lifestyle because I'm not about to change the way I live my life. It's too good, and it has taken me too long to get it that way. You see, tennis is not my whole world. It's my work. It's what I do for a living. Sure, I enjoy it and have a hell of a lot of fun playing, but it's still only part of my life. My family, my friends, and my own fulfillment are what I work *for*.

If my son wants me to spend a couple of hours shooting baskets with him, I'm going to integrate that experience into my exercise routine for that day and take credit for it. Hey, that's one of the things in life I look forward to most and I'm not about to turn him down. The day will come soon enough when he has other things he'd rather do than shoot baskets with his dad. If my wife and daughter want me to go with them on a hike through the mountains, I'll make it part of my workout for the day too. I make my lifestyle work for me.

You and I have always had a relationship of give-and-take. You keep coming out and cheering me on, and in turn, I keep giving you my best. In keeping with that tradition, I realized I needed the help of an expert to take what I do and modify it into a program that could benefit everyone. Not just any expert—the best. I enlisted the expertise of one of the finest sports medicine physicians in the world, Dr. Neil Gordon. My intent is to ensure that you get the *most* from my workout program with the *least* amount of effort and risk of injury.

Neil currently serves as the Director of Exercise Physiology at the world-renowned Cooper Institute for Aerobics Research in Dallas, Texas. In addition to his M.D. degree, he has a Ph.D. in exercise physiology and a master's degree in public health. He sits on the board of directors of the American Association of Cardiovascular and Pulmonary Rehabilitation. He also serves on the Central Research Review Committee of the American Heart Association and the Dallas board of directors of the American Heart Association. At the age of 36, Neil is already the author of over fifty scientific papers and six books on the topic of exercise and health. He has lectured extensively in the United States and abroad and is a fellow of both the American Association of Cardiovascular and Pulmonary Rehabilitation and the American College of Sports Medicine.

The first time I sat down with Neil to discuss the possibility of doing a fitness book, I had a grave concern. I wasn't sure whether or not I was the best role model for the subject. I confessed right away that my eating habits aren't always a nutritionist's dream. After all, I spend a lot of time running between hotels and airports and have two young kids who love to eat fast food.

Occasionally, when I'm not in heavy training, I also

like to enjoy a beer or two with my friends. I've never misled the public before and wanted to make it clear right from the beginning that I wouldn't start now. I may be Jimmy Connors the tennis pro on court, but off the court I'm a dad, husband, and friend. And that's the way I like it.

Neil told me that this is precisely the reason I am a good role model for the average person. In spite of all his fancy degrees, he too is a father, husband, and regular guy. Something told me that he wasn't the type of doctor who would realistically expect his patients to follow the straight and narrow 100 percent of the time. I knew I had found in Neil Gordon the right partner for this book.

Together we have created two 16-week programs— one for the person who either has never exercised regularly or who has been away from it for a significant amount of time, and one for those of you who already work out but want to take your level of fitness a step higher. Not only are these programs designed to make you fitter and healthier than you are right now, but they are intended to keep you that way forever. Regardless of how you may have neglected your body in the past, you will now be able to right the wrongs. You can regain the shape, vitality, and vigor you thought were long since gone. You can also reduce your risk for dreaded conditions such as heart attacks, high blood pressure, certain types of cancers, strokes, and diabetes.

The Jimmy Connors 16-week workouts will work for you for the same reason they work for me. They are "lifestyle-friendly." The programs aren't elaborate, don't have to take a lot of time, and don't have to be all that strenuous. Once I've shown you how to use the Connors Count℠, a clever way to listen to your own body and know the right amount of exercise for you, *you* decide how much time and effort you want to devote to working out. I'll offer suggestions and ways to ensure that you make the best decisions, but the only pressure you'll receive from my program is that which you place upon yourself. I certainly don't want to tell you how to live your life. I only want to help you live a longer, better, more productive one.

Once you're past the 16-week point, I'll show you how to stick with your program for the rest of your life. Along the way, I'll share stories with you about what happened to me when I did and didn't listen to my body. I will also give you an update on some of the latest medical discoveries in the area of health and fitness. Since I started working on this book with Neil, he has been filling my head with one study after another done by himself and other doctors around the world. While I fully appreciated the importance of all these studies, you can rest assured that the only ones you'll find here are the ones we feel could directly relate to *you*.

You should find, as I have, that there is no reason to go back to a life without exercise. The benefits of this program are too great to give up. I won't let them count me out just because I'm over 35, and I don't want you to count yourself out either. Let's get to it!

COUNTING

YOURSELF

IN

PART ONE

Don't Count Me Out

I KNEW SOMETHING extraordinary was in the wind. Call it a premonition, intuition, or whatever you want, but even before I left my home in California and headed for Flushing Meadow, New York, I had a feeling something was going to happen.

The road to the '91 U.S. Open was a long one. Since my wrist injury and surgery in 1990, I had mapped out what I thought was a realistic comeback strategy, which was to peak in New York.

The injury happened in Milan, Italy. It was early February and I was playing the first match of my first tournament of 1990. I was playing a big boomer, which is what I call the big, strong, young guys. (They all seem to be big boomers these days.) We were 5-all in the third set and 15-all in the game. I remember distinctly that it was about 9:40 in the evening when he bombed a first serve and it was long. I wasn't sure whether the linesman was going to call it, so at the very last second I tried to help it over, just in case. As I did that, I made contact with the ball and my hand just opened up and released my racquet. Immediately I looked around to a buddy of mine in the stands and said to him, "I broke my wrist." (As you might have guessed, I actually said it a little more colorfully than that.) I picked up the racquet and hit another ball. The pain was unbelievable. Every time I hit a forehand, it felt like my wrist was shattering. My body was telling me to quit and I should have stopped playing right then and there. In the back of my mind I could hear the voice of my mom, who has been my one and only coach. She too was telling me not to continue. But I did continue and lost in a tiebreaker in that third set.

As soon as the match was over, I went to the hospital in Milan. The X ray determined that the wrist wasn't broken but I couldn't move it at all. Not knowing what was wrong, they put me in a cast and sent me home. Back in the States I saw a bunch of doctors all over the country, none of whom gave me any advice I could use. I was given what seemed like a hundred different tests, including X rays, MRIs, nuclear die injected into me, and God knows what else. But all they could tell me was rest, rest, rest. So I took seven months off from tennis to rest.

By the time August came around, I was getting pretty anxious. I decided to try to play again. I made a brace for myself and wrapped the wrist real tight and went out to the court. It didn't work.

That was the week before the '90 U.S. Open, so I had to give up New York, which didn't make me too happy. I took another four or five weeks off and tried to play again in San Francisco. Things were looking up. I played two matches and won them. But just as I was beginning to think the worst was behind me, I hit a ball a little late during the third round and cringed. "Oh no," I thought. "Here we go." I had to default the match against John McEnroe, which I hated to do, but it couldn't be helped.

The next morning I went out to hit a few just to see how bad it really was, when a friend of mine, Eric Van Dillen, the guy who was running the tournament, came up to me with another man. The other guy was introduced as Dr. Jim Garrick. He said, "Jimmy, I know what's wrong with your wrist."

After almost nine months of not being told anything, I was a little leery. "Oh, jeez, Doc, are you sure?" I asked, with more than a hint of sarcasm in my voice.

He said, "I'm serious. I know what's wrong with your wrist." And then he started to explain to me that the tendon was probably severed. It made so much sense that I asked him to call Rick Scheinberg, my friend and doctor, in Santa Barbara, and explain it to him.

I rested the wrist for a couple more weeks and then went to Europe, where I was scheduled to play in two events. The wrist was so bad over there that I was actually injecting Novocain into it to relieve the pain long enough to play. That was not the brightest thing I've ever done, I don't mind telling you. Whatever the problem was, I was making it worse. Just because I didn't feel the pain doesn't mean it wasn't there.

When I returned from Europe there were more than a few messages from Rick Scheinberg. Evidently he had spoken to Dr. Garrick. I called him right away and said, "What's going on, Doc?"

"You're what's going on. You're going into the hospital at nine o'clock in the morning for wrist surgery. Look, Jimmy, you're never going to be able to play again anyway, so why don't you come in and let me try to help you at least move your wrist?"

That was a rude awakening. I was 37 years old and had been away from my regular schedule for the better part of a year. It's hard enough to keep up with the kids on the court when I'm in top form. Could this be the end of the road for me?

The next morning at nine I was in surgery. My tendon was nearly severed and the compartment that holds my wrist in place, as well as all the surrounding tissue, was gone. Dr. Scheinberg had to literally build me a new wrist.

Right after the surgery, I went through a bad time. It wasn't really a depression, but I certainly wasn't happy. I had serious concerns about whether or not I was going to be able to play again. I was confused and all I could do was wait. Over the years I've thought a lot about what I'll do when I stop playing tennis. And believe me, my family and I are going to have some good times when that happens. But these plans are being made for the time when I quit playing pro tennis. Having it taken away from me was a different matter altogether.

About two weeks later, the good Dr. Scheinberg called again and said, "OK, it's time."

I said, "Time for what? I'm in a cast. Leave me alone."

"It's time for you to get back to training, to start your program again. When your arm is well, I don't want you having even one excuse for not playing your best."

Four days a week for about five weeks, he exercised with me. It was kind of strange because he had told me to start my program again but my program consisted of some exercises that I couldn't do. So we improvised. Our goal was to improve both my aerobic and my anaerobic fitness. Both of these are crucial to me in my tennis. Aerobic or cardiorespiratory fitness, as it is often called, refers to our ability to perform moderate to vigorous levels of physical activity for prolonged periods of time in relative comfort. Without getting too technical on you, this ability is largely dependent on your body's capacity to take in oxygen from the air and process it for energy production. The more oxygen you are able to use, the more energy your muscles will be able to produce. The more energy produced, the higher the aerobic fitness level.

We'd run, jog up and down stairs, and do a variety of other aerobic activities to build up my cardiorespiratory fitness. Aerobic activities are those exercises that utilize large amounts of oxygen for energy production, and because of this, can be continued for long periods of time. At first it was kind of awkward, trying to get the right balance with one arm in a cast. Like anything else, it just took a little getting used to. Jumping rope, my favorite aerobic exercise, and, of course, my tennis were out for a while.

In contrast to aerobic activities, anaerobic exercise involves an all-out burst of energy and does not require oxygen for energy production. These kinds of activities can fatigue a person within a minute or two. When I play tennis, it is most definitely an aerobic activity. One set can take an hour or longer with virtually nonstop movement. But during any given point, I may be forced to charge to and from the net several times. Each time I do, I am performing anaerobic exercise. That's why we also included sprinting, a typical anaerobic activity, in my training.

As always, I listened carefully to my body to determine how much exercise was enough. This was especially important during my recovery period because, although I'd become quite good at knowing how much exercise I needed while healthy, I was unaccustomed to being out of the game for this much time. I knew I could easily make things worse by overdoing it.

When I got the OK to pick up the racquet again, it was almost as if I'd never played before. It reminded me of when I first taught the kids to play. I had to take it very slowly and could only practice for about five minutes a day. My wife, Patti, and son, Brett, would toss me the balls while I stood about five feet from the net. My main objective was to grip the racquet as tight as I could, bring it back, and swing through. After about ten days I moved to the service line and hit balls from there. Three weeks later, I went back to my mom and learned how to play competitive tennis all over again.

In February of '91, I was feeling so good that I said, "I gotta go play." It was a little early, and I took my knocks for the first three or four months, but I was back. I knew I could honestly say that I had done everything possible to try to keep playing. If I would have had to quit then, at least it would have been on my terms.

My plan was to take it easy and play consistently. I was going to pace myself until the U.S. Open. But the magic began a little sooner than I anticipated. I call it magic because of the aura that seemed to surround me starting at the French Open in June of 1991.

That whole spring and summer the crowds had been unbelievable, but when I got to France they were out of control. I remember waiting to be introduced on the court and hearing them chant, "Jee-mee . . . Jee-mee . . ." I couldn't figure it out. What was the big deal? Was all this attention really because I was 38 years old? Jeez, I was afraid to walk out there! I didn't want to lose in the first round and let them down.

I didn't lose in the first round. In fact, I made it into the third round against Michael Chang, which made everyone even crazier. First of all, Chang could be my son. I'm twice his age. He's known for his speed and how well he moves the ball around the court. I don't know whether the people felt sorry for me or what, but

I can tell you that Chang's parents were the only ones rooting for him in the whole place. My own energy level was so high, even I forgot that I was a 38-year-old athlete recovering from a serious injury. The truth is, I wasn't in the kind of shape I should have been to play with him at the time. I was on my way, but I wasn't quite ready. My training program was set up so that I'd peak at the end of August. I still had two months to go. But I felt like I had a chance to win, so I was giving it everything I had. What happened was, I threw my back out. It was a case of being too tired (we'd been playing for over four hours!) and trying too hard. I don't regret it, because that's my obligation to the people. When the back went out, though, it was time to leave the court. The pain was too much. I'd come too far to let something else happen to my body.

At least I quit while I was ahead. And I think I left the crowds with something to think about. Could he have won? Hey, you know, if Connors can play for four hours, maybe he could have gone on to win. I left them wondering, and to tell you the truth, I've often wondered the same thing myself.

At Wimbledon, in July, the ordinarily stoic crowd, was unusually rowdy. Again with the chanting, "Jih-mee . . . Jih-mee . . ." They cheered me royally through the third round, where I eventually lost to Derrick Rostagno. Naturally, I'd rather have won, but I felt good, was playing competitive tennis, and was having a ball on the court. I can't begin to describe how it feels to have the people behind you. I can remember a time when I was anything but the favorite.

They said I was the bad boy of tennis and I guess I was. I was often egged on by my good friend Nasty (Ilie Nastase). We were considered rebels by some. For us it was just pouring out heart and soul into every shot. But then along came Mac (John McEnroe), and all of a sudden, we didn't seem so bad anymore. Whether people like what happens when guys like us get on the court or not, they rarely want to miss it. It keeps them awake, alert, and their eyes on the court. When you're paying attention to the game, you get a lot more out of it. And whether the good people of London chose to cheer me on because they were being entertained or because they couldn't believe an "old" man like me was still out there swinging, the effect was the same. I was loving it.

So there I was having what I thought was a pretty good summer. The wrist was coming back ahead of schedule and I was playing well. I was concentrating on my tennis and my overall fitness level, and liking the results. OK, maybe I wasn't winning the big matches, but I was a contender. If I can maintain a certain standard of excellence against these young guys, I'm happy. The truth is, at 40 I don't move as well as they do, but I do other things better. I'm in there fighting and I think people are respecting that. Even when I withdrew in the third round at the French Open and lost in round three at Wimbledon, I felt encouraged. They were calling me "the comeback kid." For me, the fun was back in the game again and my playing seemed to grip the public. I was being stopped everywhere I went by people wishing me luck. My family and friends couldn't have been more supportive. I was ready for Flushing Meadows.

One night late in August, I was sitting around after dinner with the family, talking about the upcoming tournament. Patti was saying things like "Just go out and play your best and don't worry if you don't win. You're still recuperating, everybody knows that." I understood what she was trying to say. Like any good wife, she wanted to keep me from being disappointed.

My son, Brett, who is 12 going on 40, was kind of quiet during the conversation, which really isn't like him. Finally, I said, "Brett, how about you? Do you think I'm ready for New York?"

I'll never forget his answer. "I don't know, Dad. I think you've got a bad case of third-round-itis. You do OK till the third round and then you lose. I think you should just try to get past the third round this time."

Ouch. I wanted to say to him, "Hey, what's the deal, Bretter? I'm your dad, give me a break." But he was right. I hadn't made it past the third round in a long time. When everyone else was telling me what they thought I wanted to hear, my son told me what I *needed* to hear. He spoke to me like a true friend.

As I was about to board the plane, Brett's final words were "You know what you've got to do, Dad."

His words, innocent though they may have been, struck a nerve. I knew I'd do *anything* to get past the third round of that tournament. Like I said before, motivation comes from a lot of different places.

There was something in the air from the moment I arrived at Flushing Meadows just a couple of days prior to my 39th birthday. I usually don't like to know my draw in advance. I never have. I figure, what's the point? I'm going to play the best tennis I know how no matter who my opponent is. I don't need to worry about adjusting my game to suit the other guy. But about two days before the tournament began, someone came up to me and said, "Hey, Connors, you play McEnroe!"

And I thought, "Yes! My pal John. Now that will be fun." Then they told me it was Patrick McEnroe. And in a way I felt, "Jeez, I've gone through all these great matches with John over the years and now I'm playing his little brother. Next I'll be playing his son."

I had practiced with Patrick and knew he was playing well. I was also aware that because he was a New Yorker, there would probably be a good crowd. Someone from the tournament came to me and said, "We want to play you at night because it's Connors and McEnroe."

Tennis fans, by nature, usually prefer afternoon matches. I guess the officials thought having Patrick and me play at night might bring a few more people out. So I said, "Fine, play me at night."

Before I went down to the court, I called home for a quick pep talk from the family. My seven-year-old daughter, Aubree, answered the phone. "Daddy," she said, "I know you're going to at least win your first match because I put a quarter in the wishing well and that's what I wished for."

And I said, "Great! If it works you'll have to put fifty cents in tomorrow."

"Maybe I want you *home* tomorrow, Dad," she replied. God bless little girls.

I don't think anyone expected the four-hour-and-twenty-minute match that went on until 1:30 in the morning. Least of all me. Patrick should have taken me in straight sets, and he almost did. I was down two sets when more than half the stadium decided to call it a night. Those who remained moved down real close. It was like playing in a large boxing arena. What the crowd lacked in size, however, it made up for in volume. I was struggling badly in the beginning of the third set and they sort of willed me through it. When Patrick made an error and I took advantage of it, the fans became very emotional. So did I. From that point on I couldn't do anything wrong—the crowd wouldn't let me. As I walked off the court, energized from the victory, I could still hear the people clapping and cheering my name. I was overwhelmed.

Later that night, long after the stadium had cleared, I came back and strolled around all by myself. In the stillness of the deserted court, I recalled the magic of the hours before. I was surprised at how much this night meant to me. I mean, it *was* only the first round. In years past I wouldn't have felt this kind of emotion until after I'd won the entire tournament, or not at all.

The next day I was pretty tired, but I went out to hit a few just to keep from stiffening up. When I got out to the court, there were about 2,000 spectators standing around and about twenty newspeople with cameras. I thought, "What's going on? Is Becker coming out or something?" It really never dawned on me that they were there to see me. When I found out, well, it felt pretty wonderful. But I remember thinking, "These people must really think I'm old. They never made this much of a fuss over me before!"

My second-round opponent was Michiel Schapers. Again, they scheduled us to play at night, hoping, I'm sure, for a repeat of the drama of the McEnroe match. Evidently, the fans wanted it too, because the crowd of 19,582 was a record breaker for the night session. I was three days shy of turning 39 years old and I think the people wanted to see me prove that I hadn't lost it—for their sake as much as mine. They needed me to show them that being almost 40 was not a detriment.

I guess I showed them, but not in the manner they hoped for. I took Schapers in three sets, the total length of the match was one hour and forty-two minutes. I didn't mind having an easy time of it at all. The only thing that mattered was that I won, and I did. Now it was time for the third round.

I was feeling kind of badly that Patti and the kids weren't there with me. I didn't get married and have children to leave them at home. I really miss them when I'm gone, and I was missing them more than ever in New York because of all the excitement. But Brett and Aubree had just started the school year and it would have been too disruptive to take them out. Patti needed to be with them. We made a deal that if I got to the finals, they would all come to New York for the weekend. I talked to Brett that morning before he left for school. "I'm playing my third round today, Bretter. What do you say?"

"OK, Dad," he said. "You try to win it and I'll call Mom from school to find out what happened."

I won the match against Karel Novacek in three straight sets. When I called Patti afterward, she told me Brett had called her five times from school. She was watching on TV and gave him the play-by-play. Winning that match was the highlight of the tournament for me, and that's saying a lot, because the whole tournament was like a dream.

I won my next round against Aaron Krickstein in a grueling four-hour-and-forty-one-minute match and I took Haarhuis in the quarterfinals in a match that lasted just under four hours. For this reason, not only was it important that my tennis was back to competitive level, but I could never have lasted through those matches if my level of fitness wasn't back as well. It was hotter than hell in New York and the humidity was a killer. People say I'm still around because I have a lot of heart, but I know all the heart in the world couldn't have helped me if I wasn't physically fit. I owe much of my success to my workout program.

I lost in the semifinals to Jim Courier. Although I probably went beyond most people's expectations of what they thought I could do, I was disappointed. I may have accepted the fact that I won't win every tournament anymore, but that doesn't mean that I don't *want* to win and that I don't *try* to win. Still, I came to play good tennis and that's what I did. All in all, I had a great tournament.

Of course, there were a lot of variables that entered into the picture. Andre Agassi lost in the first round and

Boris Becker lost in the third. If I would have beaten Becker and Agassi in the tournament, my ranking would have jumped even higher. So it was good that they didn't win and it was bad that they didn't win. But I can't go back and worry about that now. The excitement of that tournament was beyond belief for me.

Anyway, it was almost as if I *had* won. I don't know how I could have been treated any better. Even when I lost, the crowd was on their feet, yelling, "Nupe it, Jimmy! Nupe it!" You know, I waited twenty years for a tournament like that. It was a payback for all the blood, sweat, and tears of matches gone by. I don't think there will ever be another one like it. Most people don't even remember that Stefan Edberg ended up winning the whole deal. At the end of the tournament I heard him talking to the press. He said, "Connors may have received all the attention here this week, but in years to come when people look at that trophy sitting at Flushing Meadows, it will be my name they see engraved as the winner of the 1991 U.S. Open."

I just looked at him, smiled, and said, "That may be true, my friend. But *my* name will have appeared five times *before* yours."

2

Being Fit. What Does It Mean?

BEING FIT is one of those phrases that mean something different to everyone. And whatever it means to you today may not be what it means a year from now or five years from now. There is no right or wrong definition of being fit.

Right now my idea of being fit is having the ability to play good, competitive tennis for five hours at a time with guys half my age. That is my need today. When I decide to retire from professional tennis my needs will be totally different. I'll always want to look good, that's a given. I'm as vain as anyone else and I want to fit into these same size clothes for as long as I can. For me, that will always take a certain amount of exercise because I have a strong propensity to gain weight. The one year I didn't concentrate on my fitness I gained 35 pounds! I don't intend to let that happen again.

More important than how I look is having the ability to enjoy my life to the fullest. I want to be able to ski, run, hike, or engage in any other activity with my wife and kids, and my kids' families when the time comes. If I can't participate because I'm not fit enough, that would be a terrible loss to me.

The most important reason for me to maintain a certain level of fitness, however, is to prevent the onset of those diseases that are associated with physical inactivity. Now that I've turned 40, I'd be a fool not to think about what I can do to prolong my life. I've learned that I can dramatically decrease the risk of heart attack, high blood pressure, diabetes, and many other dreaded illnesses with even a minimal amount of exercise. The level at which I exercise today is part of my job. When I give up tennis, what I do won't be nearly as tough or as time-consuming, but I'll always include some sort of fitness plan in my life. I haven't worked this hard for this long to lose it all to a sickness that could have been prevented.

There are two major categories of fitness: *performance-related* and *health-related* (see Figure 2-1). *Performance-related fitness* is for those who want to be able to excel in competitive athletics. Their workout routines are strenuous, the goal being to get their bodies into the kind of shape where they can call on them to perform at top level anytime, anywhere.

Health-related fitness is for those who are not interested in physical competition but want to reach and

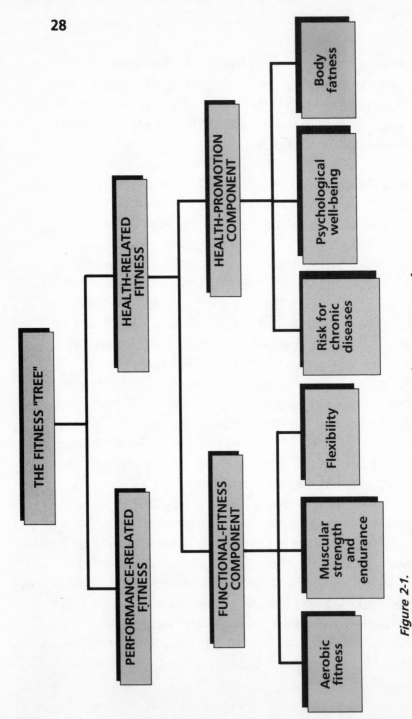

Figure 2-1.
The fitness "tree"—the major categories and components of fitness.

maintain a degree of fitness that allows them to get the most out of life. Within this health-related category are two components: the *functional-fitness* component and the *health-promotion* component. *Functional fitness* is defined in terms of being a participant, having the ability to do the activities you enjoy or would like to enjoy with vigor and enthusiasm. For me, functional fitness means being able to put in 45 minutes of training, four hours of hard-core tennis practice, working in the office for a couple of hours on my various business deals, and then having enough energy to play with my children and take my wife out the same night. Down the road it may mean having the energy to put in a 30-minute workout, take care of my business, work out in the yard, play with my grandchildren, and take my wife out at night. The point is, we should not be forced to give up anything that makes us happy just because we age, nor should we be afraid to try something new just because we're getting older.

The *health-promotion* component deals with diminishing the risk of disease. I can't stress enough the importance of the health component. Nothing you can achieve, buy, or love is going to bring you fulfillment if you're not around to enjoy it. Those of us fortunate enough to have our health have an obligation not to abuse it.

This book targets health-related fitness. It is the area of fitness most people can relate to and want to explore. Throughout the coming chapters, as I talk more about health-related fitness, I will speak of the functional-fitness component as exercising for fitness and the health-promotion component as exercising for health. Although I have been an advocate of performance-related fitness for most of my life, I can assure you this is only because my job demands it. My needs will soon be similar to yours and I'll have neither the reason nor the desire to push myself as hard as I do now.

I believe everyone owes it to themselves and those who love them to be actively involved in living. But we can't become actively involved without preparation. If you don't have the energy to participate, you simply can't do it. When you are uncomfortable with the way you look, your desire to participate is also understandably lessened. Before I lost those 35 pounds I didn't want anyone to see me, considerably limiting my choice of activities. And if you're sick or injured, the energy you have must be spent getting better. Yes, the body must be conditioned to take on the opponent of life.

I don't think there is a person alive who hasn't heard that exercise is beneficial to the body, to the mind, and to the spirit. Yet Neil tells me that 50 percent of those who begin a workout program drop out within three to six months of the day they started. Available research supports the idea that incorporating exercise into a sedentary lifestyle is a more difficult behavioral change than many others. I'm not going to tell you that if you're not used to working out, it's going to be easy at first. I wouldn't kid you about that. But I can promise you that each workout will get easier.

I'm no expert in psychology, but I have a theory. It has to do with the difference between *self-control* and *self-discipline.* Self-control is about keeping yourself from doing something you want to do. For example, if I want to indulge in a big piece of fudge cake, but decide against it for the sake of my diet or health, I have exhibited self-control. If, on the other hand, I wake up in the morning feeling like lounging around in bed all day rather than going out to the court, but make myself do it anyway, I have exhibited self-discipline. Although it is important to have both self-control and self-discipline at times in our lives, I believe self-discipline is often the more difficult concept to put into action.

Maybe it has to do with Newton's law of motion. It is harder to make yourself do something you don't want to do than to keep yourself from doing something you do want to do. That's why I believe most people drop out of their exercise program.

My objective is twofold. First, to convince you beyond a shadow of a doubt that your life will be more fulfilling if you exercise regularly, and second, to provide you with a program so lifestyle-friendly and effective that once you make the decision to start, you'll never want to stop again. Whatever being fit means to you is OK with me. If it means fitting into a certain size of clothing, being able to keep up with your kids, preventing the onset of a disease, or having the ability to run a couple of miles—so be it. No matter what the specifics may be of your personal definition of being fit, there is one thing we must agree on before you begin. Life is not a spectator sport.

3

What's in It for You?

PEOPLE HAVE BEEN TALKING about the virtues of physical activity for centuries. Literally. In fact, I believe it was Hippocrates, the fifth-century-B.C. Greek doctor, who stated so eloquently, "All parts of the body which have a function, if used in moderation and exercised in labors in which each is accustomed, become thereby healthy, well developed, and age more slowly; but if unused and left idle they become liable to disease, defective in growth, and age quickly." Translation? Use it or lose it.

Yes, if you've heard it once, you've heard it a million times. Exercise is good for you. Big deal. I understand spinach is good for you too, but simply hearing the words "It's good for you" wouldn't motivate me to eat the stuff. Besides, there are choices other than spinach that will provide me with the same benefits.

No, if I weren't already motivated to exercise, I would want to know exactly what's in it for me before I committed the time and energy. I would want to know specifically what benefits I'd get from my efforts. "It's good for you" just doesn't do it for me and probably not for you either. So let's find out what you will get from having a regular fitness routine.

Remember, throughout this book we are talking about health-related fitness rather than performance-related fitness. Health-related fitness is for those of you who are interested in the prevention of diseases related to inactivity and/or taking your current degree of physical ability to the next level, rather than preparing your body for top-level physical competition. I realize that many people want to exercise for the sole purpose of looking good, and that's fine. If this is your only reason for starting my workout program, I have some news for you. Whether you like it or not, you will improve your health and raise the level of your physical ability in the process. The same applies for those of you who begin this program with the intent to prevent disease and heighten your level of physical ability. Chances are, by the end of 16 weeks, you'll see a marked improvement in the way you look. That's the way it goes.

EXERCISING TO IMPROVE FITNESS

In order to appreciate the benefits of exercise you must be familiar with the three main types of functional fitness: aerobic fitness (which I discussed with you in Chapter 1), muscular strength and endurance, and flexibility. A balanced fitness program should target all three.

Aerobic or *cardiorespiratory fitness,* as you know, refers to your ability to perform moderate to vigorous levels of physical activity for prolonged periods of time in relative comfort. But did you know that up until 1968, if you had looked up the word "aerobic" in the dictionary, it would have been defined as an adjective meaning "growing in air or oxygen"? It was commonly used to describe bacteria that needed oxygen to live. In 1968, however, Dr. Ken Cooper coined the term "aerobics" as a noun, meaning those types of exercises that can be done for long periods of time because they utilize large amounts of oxygen for energy production.

Muscular strength refers to the maximum force that can be generated by a specific muscle or group of muscles. Think of it as the ability to lift, push, pull, or carry weighty objects. Even simple things we take for granted, like picking up a bag of groceries, require muscular strength. Parents depend on muscular strength every time they pick up their child. Quite often kids will ask to be picked up and put down many times throughout a given time period. This requires not only muscular strength but *muscular endurance.* I remember many a trip to Disneyland when the kids couldn't decide whether they wanted to run through the park or be held. Patti and I would take turns picking them up and holding them for what seemed like hours at a time. This takes both muscular strength and muscular endurance (and more than a little patience).

Flexibility is being able to move a joint through its full range of motion. Every time you bend over to tie your shoe, reach up to get something off a shelf, or stretch to change a light bulb, you are exhibiting flexibility. On the court, it is flexibility that allows me to get those overheads and reach up to hit a strong serve.

It should be pretty clear that we need a certain amount of aerobic fitness, strength, and flexibility to function normally throughout the day. I don't know how you feel about it, but functioning normally isn't good enough for me. I want more. And with a minimal amount of effort all of us can get much more. Neil has filled me in on all kinds of studies that show clearly that moderate exercise done regularly can greatly improve our level of fitness, which will, in turn, dramatically improve the quality of our lives. I want you to know about some of the things that came out of these studies. Look, after you've been on my program for a couple of months, you *are* going to see a big difference in the way you look and feel. When people ask you about the change, you'll be able to tell them not only what you did but why it worked.

Staying a Participant A balanced fitness program plays an important role in keeping us from the state where our cardiorespiratory fitness, strength, and flexibility are so poor that we can no longer take care of ourselves. This dreaded place has been termed the "disability zone." Staying out of the disability zone is as important to some as staying alive. I know it is to me. *But we must prepare now.* Experts believe that an exercise program such as the ones described in this book can keep us participating actively in life for decades longer than we could by being sedentary. (See Figure 3-1.) You see, most people are under the assumption that age causes disability and fatigue. The truth is that in many cases *inactivity* causes disability and fatigue. I think this is great news because if disability were a biological symptom of aging, there would be nothing we could do about it. Knowing that being active will *keep* us active should make us less afraid, and more accepting of the inevitable aging process. Hey, I don't mind getting older, I just don't want to look or act older than I feel. And I don't feel old.

Elevated Cardiorespiratory Fitness Cardiorespiratory fitness is usually greatest between the ages of 15 and 30, decreasing progressively as the years pass. By age 65, cardiorespiratory fitness is typically 40 percent less than in young adults. But the experts say that cardiorespiratory fitness increases by anywhere from 15 to 30 percent with an appropriate fitness program. And, while there is a 9 percent reduction in cardiorespiratory fitness per decade after the age of 30 in people who are sedentary, there is less than a 5 percent reduction per decade in people who are physically active. This means that not only can you turn back the hands of time and regain the fitness you enjoyed when you were younger but you can slow down the aging process!

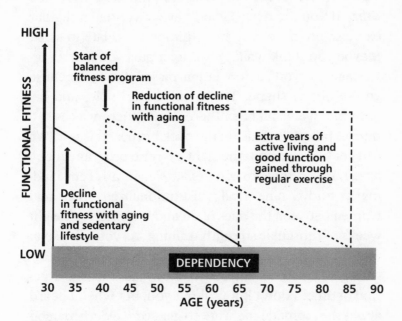

Figure 3-1.
Gaining extra years of active living through regular exercise. This figure shows that a balanced exercise program, such as the Jimmy Connors workout program, can play an important role both in increasing your fitness and reducing its decline with age. Such benefits prolong your "active" lifespan by delaying the onset of dependency—that is, the state where your functional fitness is so poor that you are no longer able to take care of yourself. (Adapted from W. Evans and I. H. Rosenberg, *Biomarkers: The 10 Determinants of Aging You Can Control.* New York: Simon & Schuster, 1991.)

You Can Reap the Benefits No Matter When You Start If you are over 35 and have never had a regular exercise program, you may think it's too late to start. Maybe you think waiting this long puts you at a disadvantage or you're too embarrassed to try because you're out of shape. This is understandable, and believe me, we've all been there. But if there was ever a time to put your pride on the back burner, this is it. We can get benefits from the right exercise program at any age. Look at this amazing example. In a recent landmark study, nine frail, institutionalized men and women between the ages of 86 and 96 undertook eight weeks of muscular strength training. As you can see in Figure 3-2, the volunteers showed an average of a staggering 174 percent improvement in just this short period of time! I don't know about you, but when I heard about this, it made me want to get every elderly person I know on a fitness plan. To think that even a 96-year-old person can improve the quality of their life with moderate effort is very exciting to me. Imagine what it could do for you.

EXERCISING TO IMPROVE HEALTH

Just as there are three main types of functional fitness, there are also three main aspects to the health-promotion component of health-related fitness. They are: your risk for chronic diseases, your degree of body fatness, and your psychological well-being. Let's take a closer look at how a balanced program of regular exer-

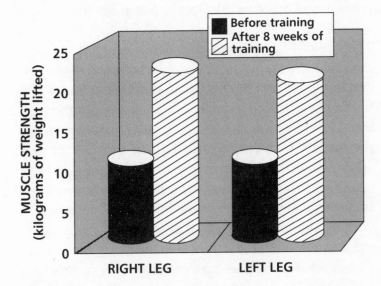

Figure 3-2.
You can reap the benefits no matter when you start. In this study, conducted by researchers from Tufts University, Boston, nine volunteers between the ages of 86 and 96 years increased their leg strength by an average of 174 percent with eight weeks of strength training. (Adapted from M. A. Fiatarone et al., "High-Intensity Strength Training in Nonagenarians: Effects on Skeletal Muscle," *Journal of the American Medical Association,* 1990, 263:3029–3034.)

cise favorably affects each of these aspects. I'm not going to discuss these benefits in order of importance because there is no particular benefit that stands out among the others. Each will hold its own unique importance as it is needed throughout a lifetime.

The Weight-Loss Factor Just about everyone I know talks about wanting to lose weight now and then. Evidently, about half the people in the United States feel the same way. Neil tells me that 37 percent of the men and 52 percent of the women in this country consider themselves overweight. In fact, 20 percent of our adults *are* actually overweight to the extent that their health and longevity are compromised. People become overweight when too many calories are consumed in the diet and too few are used up during physical activity. In most cases, caloric restriction combined with regular exercise is the most effective way of reaching and maintaining an ideal body weight. This is not new news. We all know that exercise burns calories, which aids in weight control. What many people don't realize, however, is that the benefits of exercise go way beyond the burning of extra calories while you're working out. This is why most experts rate regular exercise as the most important factor of an effective weight-control program. (See Figure 3-3, p. 42.)

Burn Calories While You Sleep Burn calories while you sleep? Are they kidding? Nope. Muscle cells are metabolically active and burn calories even while you are at rest. The more muscle you have, the more calories you will burn throughout the course of a day. To me that's as good a reason as any for replacing fat with muscle. Unfortunately, when you go on a diet, you lose both fat and muscle. What you want to do, obviously, is minimize muscle loss while maximizing fat loss. A balanced fitness program consisting of aerobic activity and strength training will do the job for you. Of course, there are other, less scientific reasons for replacing fat with muscle. You'll lose the flab, your body will be firmer and more shapely, and your clothes will look better on you.When I put on that extra weight a few years ago it was because I stopped working out regularly. My eating habits didn't change much, although with more time on my hands, I probably snacked a little more often. Almost immediately after I got back into my program, the weight started coming off.

Exercise Minimizes the Plateaus Anyone who has ever gone on a diet knows the frustration of hitting a plateau, those places on the way down where your weight seems to get stuck for a period of time. No matter how little you eat, the scale won't budge. It seems to have a mind of its own. These times can defeat a person to the point where the diet becomes history altogether. Hang on. Exercise can help there too. Typically, when you go on a diet, your body attempts to adapt to the reduced intake of calories by slowing down the speed at which it burns them. This is your body's way of conserving energy when it senses deprivation.

Afraid of being starved, the body puts everything

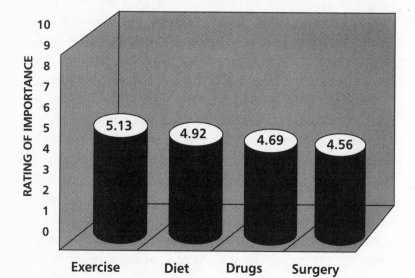

Figure 3-3.
How the experts rate the effectiveness of obesity treatments. North American experts in the field of obesity treatment were asked to rate the importance of various weight-loss interventions on a scale from 0 (not important) to 10 (extremely important). As can be seen, of the four interventions shown above, exercise was rated to be of most importance. (Adapted from G. A. Bray et al., "A Survey of Opinions of Obesity Experts on the Causes and Treatment of Obesity," *American Journal of Clinical Nutrition,* 1992, 55:151S–154S.)

into slow motion in order to save energy, probably thinking you'll blow your diet before it runs out completely. It is during this slow-motion period that the body gets stuck at a certain weight. Studies show that a single bout of exercise often forces the body to continue burning calories at a faster rate for several hours. And when done regularly, exercise also helps prevent—or at least minimize—the natural decline in the speed at which your body burns calories when on a diet. This, in turn, helps you to lose the weight more easily than you would by dieting alone. I think that's a damn good reason for exercising. I'd probably still be carrying around that extra 35 pounds of mine if I depended only on my diet to lose it.

Exercise Reduces the Risk of Chronic Disease Not only does a sedentary lifestyle cause emotional, psychological, and physical discomfort; other serious health risks are also associated with it. The human body was made to move. When deprived of movement it often rebels by developing potentially devastating illnesses such as coronary heart disease, high blood pressure, osteoporosis (brittle bone disease), diabetes, strokes, and certain types of cancer.

You probably already know that coronary heart disease, which causes heart attacks, is the leading killer in the United States and in many other countries as well. It accounts for about 28 percent of the 2.1 million annual deaths in this country alone. In a major study reported by researchers from the Centers for Disease Control in Atlanta, it was proven that inactivity was just as likely to cause a heart attack as smoking, high blood pressure, and elevated cholesterol. Regular exercise can reduce your risk of dying from coronary heart disease by almost 50 percent. If that information isn't enough reason to start a workout program, I can't imagine what is.

The Mind Game They say that exercise is as good for you mentally and emotionally as it is physically. I believe it. Whenever I have an important decision to make, the first thing I want to know is, can it wait? If it's not a matter of life or death, I prefer to go out to the tennis court for a while and hit some balls before giving an answer one way or another. It's not that I think about the decision I have to make while I'm out there. On the contrary, I prefer only to think about the tennis while I'm on the court. But I have found that after a little workout my mind is so much clearer and I'm so much more relaxed that I almost always make a wiser choice. Many people feel the same way. I don't know if anyone has ever done a study on this, but I'll bet that as many people exercise regularly just for the feeling of satisfaction they get *after* their workout as those who exercise for the feeling they get during it. Remember back in Chapter 2 when I talked about the difference between self-control and self-discipline? Though it may seem overwhelming at the time, making myself get out there and physically do something gives me a sense of accomplishment. I'm proud of myself for having done it. That's good for my ego. I've found that feeding my ego with a sense of accomplishment does a hell of a lot more for me in the long run than feeding my face with chocolate cake.

There are medical studies that back up my theory. Exercise triggers the release of endorphins, the hormones produced by the pituitary gland in the brain. Endorphins have a morphine-like effect that temporarily relieves minor aches and pains as well as providing us with an all-is-right-in-the-world feeling that lasts for several hours after exercise. This sense of well-being may help us to handle life's everyday trials and tribulations (otherwise known as stress) with a much better attitude. Besides, there is no better "tired" for me than the tired I feel from a good workout.

A Little Goes a Long Way Not only is it important that you know exercise is good for you; by now you should understand *why*. Still, if the thought of beginning a tough, rigorous workout program is enough to send you back under the covers, don't despair. There is more good news. Even a moderate amount of exercise will help save your life. It's true. A recent study performed by Neil's buddies at the Cooper Institute for Aerobics Research in Dallas, which tracked about 13,000 men and women for approximately eight years, proved this enlightening concept. (See Figure 3-4.) The people in the study were divided into three groups according to their level of aerobic fitness. (Participants were tested on a treadmill to determine their level.) One group consisted of the least fit individuals, the next group contained those who were moderately fit, and the third group included only those with a high level of fitness.

The people in the moderate-fitness group were found to be at a far lower risk of dying during the study period than those in the unfit group. But the difference in risk of premature death between the moderate- and the high-fitness groups was not nearly as dramatic. The moral to this story is that you don't have to be a top-notch fitness freak to get the benefits of regular exercise. A modest exercise program, like either of the ones in this book, can be performed by almost anyone at any age and will tremendously improve the length and quality of their life. To me, this is pretty exciting news. I mean, why exercise to save your life if the amount of exercise you do makes you feel like you want to die?

I don't think anyone can quarrel with the idea that regular exercise, even if it's only a modest amount, does us a world of good. Still, there are certain risks I feel obligated to discuss. Occasionally we do hear about great athletes who meet a tragic and untimely death while exercising. The thought of dropping dead during a workout is a chilling thought for anyone. Studies have proven, however, that it wasn't the exercise itself that was the problem for these athletes, but rather the combination of strenuous exercise and a preexisting heart condition.

As part of my program, Neil and I will tell you how to determine whether you are at risk for sudden cardiac death during exercise, whether you should see a doctor before starting either one of my workouts, and

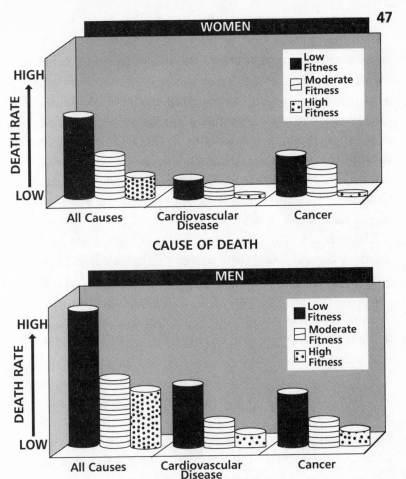

Figure 3-4.
Moderate aerobic fitness levels provide major health benefits. This figure summarizes the findings of a landmark eight-year study of 10,224 men and 3,124 women conducted by researchers from the Cooper Institute for Aerobics Research. Men and women who were only moderately fit were at a far lower risk of dying during the study period than those who were unfit. Although the highly fit study participants were at an even lower risk, the difference between them and the moderately fit individuals was not very striking. (Adapted from S. N. Blair et al., "Physical Fitness and All-Cause Mortality: A Prospective Study of Healthy Men and Women," *Journal of the American Medical Association*, 1989, 262:2395–2401.)

what you can do to minimize the risk of having a heart attack during exercise. I can assure you of one thing. You are much more likely to die because of factors associated with *not* exercising than you are because you did exercise. A little later in the book, I'm going to present you with a tool that will help you listen to your body. This tool used in conjunction with the Connors Count will minimize your risk of experiencing any sort of problem while working out.

There is also the chance that you could get injured during exercise. Hey, it happens. I've certainly experienced my share of injuries. Before you start, I will share with you precautions you can take to minimize dramatically the risk of injury. Remember, my goal is to help you improve the quality of your life, not give you more to worry about.

The last potential problem I want to discuss is becoming obsessed with exercise. I'm sure you probably know people who eat, breathe, and sleep exercise. As with any of the good things in life, there are those who will take it too far. Besides running the risk of serious injury, these people have a tendency to bore all those around them, and probably even bore themselves. They miss the point of exercise altogether. Exercise is intended to help enhance the other aspects of their lives. I like to think of exercise in the same way I think of brushing my teeth. I do it every day because if I didn't, the consequences would be terrible and because my mouth feels so good when I've finished. When I quit tennis, I will still work out regularly—as part of my preventive health care, to enhance my appearance, and to make me feel better. Just as I don't discuss the fine art of teeth brushing with everyone I meet, my workouts will be something I do for me.

Now that I've discussed the potential risks of regular exercise, you should know that virtually all of these risks are far greater for those, like myself, who are into performance-related fitness. Health-related fitness, which is the subject of this book, has far fewer risks attached to it. If you are starting one of my programs either to ward off disease or to take your degree of fitness to a higher level, there is no need to worry. I'll be with you every step of the way.

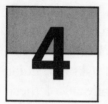

4

The Million-Dollar Question: How Much Is Enough?

THROUGHOUT THIS BOOK, I've used terms like "modest exercise," "moderate exercise," and "minimum effort." If I were you, I'd want me to quit being so evasive and explain exactly what I mean. Is it really possible to get all the benefits necessary to improve your health and/or fitness level without killing yourself? You bet it is. And I'm going to show you how.

There are three major types of exercise: *aerobic exercise* to improve cardiorespiratory fitness, *weight* or *resistance training* to improve muscular strength and endurance, and *stretching* exercises to improve flexibility. Although a balanced fitness program should contain all three, how much you need of each one differs considerably. Because of this, we are going to take a look at the three types of exercise separately in this chapter. And in doing so, you are going to see two names you probably thought would never come together, Borg and Connors, team up to teach you *how to listen to your body* and discover the answer to that million-dollar question, how much exercise is enough?

CARDIORESPIRATORY FITNESS

Before we talk about strength training and stretching, we should examine aerobic exercise. In my opinion, aerobic exercise is the most crucial of the three. It has provided me with the energy to make it to the top in professional tennis and is what will ultimately improve your health and your level of fitness.

Through many years of experience and a great deal of trial and error (hopefully a little more trial than error), I know exactly how much aerobic exercise I need in order to play top-level tennis. I use each tournament as a measuring stick in gauging how fit I am, and adjust my workouts accordingly. Fortunately, you don't have to play a guessing game. When it comes to health-related fitness, enough research studies have been done now to eliminate the process of trial and error. We now know within a certain range how much aerobic exercise is needed for health-related fitness. Once you get into this range, you can adjust the amount to meet your own needs.

Improvements in health-related fitness, either your level of fitness or the state of your health, are mostly related to the *amount of energy* you expend (or the number of calories you burn) during exercise each week. Although any increase of energy output above a sedentary person's current level will probably be of some benefit, a certain minimum level of weekly expenditure must be reached in order to get a substantial benefit. This minimum level, according to the American Heart Association, is a weekly output of energy during exercise totaling 700 calories.

As you increase your energy expenditure or the number of calories you burn throughout the week, the amount of benefit you get for your efforts will increase as well. However, and this is important, the benefits plateau at about 2,000 calories. Beyond that point no additional benefits are likely to occur. (However, those competitive athletes who exercise to obtain a performance-related fitness level will probably receive additional benefit after 2,000 calories.) For health-related fitness, the American Heart Association recommends not less than 700 or more than 2,000 calories burned during exercise per week. So now you know there is a limit. No one expects you to hop till you drop.

Weekly energy expended during exercise depends largely on four factors: the type of exercise, the frequency of the exercise, the intensity of the exercise, and the duration of the exercise. As I've already discussed, aerobic exercise is a far more efficient way of burning calories than anaerobic exercise, because energy expenditure is directly related to how much oxygen your working muscles use during exercise. You can do aerobic exercise for longer periods of time, allowing you to expend far more energy, without becoming excessively tired.

The next three factors are entwined in a concept called FIT. FIT is an acronym for Frequency, Intensity, and Time. Frequency refers to how often you exercise. Intensity refers to how hard you exercise. Time refers to how long you exercise.

Frequency Ideally, you should exercise 5 days each week. Exercising 6 or 7 days per week will not necessarily result in greater health-related fitness, but may increase your risk for injury. On the other hand, working out 2 or fewer days per week does not result in any great improvements. To compromise, you should exercise a minimum of 3 days each week.

Space your workouts as evenly as possible throughout the 7-day period. For example, if you're a 3-day-a-weeker, rather than exercise on Monday, Tuesday, and Wednesday, you'd be better off exercising on Monday, Wednesday, and Friday. Although it isn't of much importance from a fitness standpoint, it does make a difference from a health standpoint.

You see, exercise delivers part of its health benefits much the same way that medicine delivers its benefits. Let's say you have just injured yourself and your doc has told you to take some medication (Nuprin, for example) for a few days to reduce pain and inflammation. As good a medication as it is, the anti-inflammatory effects will only last for a short period of time before they begin to wear off. This is why your doctor may tell you to take the medication every 4 to 6 hours.

If you wait too long before "Nupin' it" the second time, all the previous medication will have worn off and the inflammation may be back in full force. The same applies to exercise. If you abstain from exercise for more than 2 or 3 days at a time, you will lose some of the health benefits you got from your previous workout.

Time When the purpose is to optimize health-related fitness, workouts usually last anywhere from 15 to 60 minutes (20 to 40 minutes being ideal for most people). A workout involving 15 to 60 minutes of *continuous* aerobic activity has long been considered the right amount of time needed to receive the most benefit. But recently another option has proven to be equally effective. This research finding is a real breakthrough and contradicts most of what we've been taught in the past.

Three 10-minute exercise sessions *spread throughout* the day appear to do as much for you as one 30-minute session. (See Figure 4-1.) In other words, you can split the aerobic portion of your workout into several shorter bouts of exercise if you choose. Some people like to do their workout in one shot, preferring to limit their shower time and/or changing-of-clothes time to a minimum. Others see it as great news. When I'm in training for a tournament, I often capitalize on this, dividing my day's tennis practice into a morning session and an afternoon session. Because I don't get as tired, I'm able to concentrate better during these shorter practice sessions and it makes me feel as if I'm getting twice the benefit. I've seen the way some of the

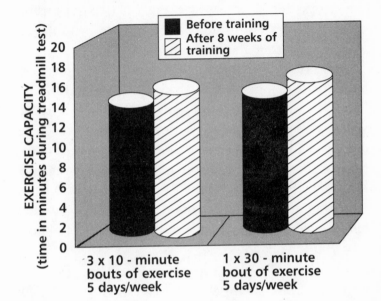

Figure 4-1.
Comparison between short and long bouts of exercise. In an eight-week study conducted by researchers from Stanford University, the effectiveness of three 10-minute exercise sessions spread throughout the day was compared with that of one 30-minute session. In both cases, study participants trained 5 days per week at a moderate intensity. Aerobic fitness, measured with treadmill testing, increased by approximately 12 percent with both the short and long exercise sessions. (Adapted from R. F. DeBusk et al., "Training Effects of Long Versus Short Bouts of Exercise in Healthy Subjects," *American Journal of Cardiology,* 1990, 65:1010–1013.)

other guys on the circuit practice. They stay out on the court for hours sometimes right before a match. Whatever works for them is great, but I like to get on the court, take care of business, and get the hell off. It's what keeps the game fresh for me.

If you're just beginning a program, 10 minutes can be a lot less intimidating than 30. You may think, "Hey, I can handle ten minutes of anything!" Maybe you have certain time restrictions that seem easier to manage with several shorter workouts. The benefits of this concept will become even more obvious in the next chapter, where I teach how to work shorter bouts of exercise into daily life. No matter which time duration best fills your needs, it should be comforting to know that you have a choice.

Intensity Until fairly recently, exercise enthusiasts, including myself, were under the impression that the only effective exercise was tough exercise. We thought that unless you felt a significant amount of pain during the process, the benefits were not worth talking about. As I'm sure you've heard by now, this type of thinking is passé. There is no need to exercise to the point of pain in order to get positive results. Quite the contrary.

Let me tell you about one study that helps prove the theory that a little goes a long way when it comes to exercise. The purpose of the study was to determine how important exercise intensity is when it comes to both health and fitness.

The subjects for the study were 102 sedentary women between the ages of 20 and 40. Each woman was randomly placed in one of four groups. The first group remained sedentary. The other three groups each walked 3 miles 5 days per week. One of them walked slowly, at a pace of 20 minutes per mile; another walked briskly, at 15 minutes per mile; and the final group walked fast, at 12 minutes per mile. After six months, all four groups were reevaluated. Fitness levels did not improve in the group that remained sedentary. In fact, they decreased slightly. As you can see in Figure 4-2, cardiorespiratory fitness levels increased in direct proportion to the walking speed in the other three groups. The faster or more intensely they walked, the higher their cardiorespiratory fitness improvement.

However, and this is the part I think will surprise you, the same was not true in measuring the benefits of intensity in relation to health. You see, the risk of heart disease decreased in the slow-walking group to about the same degree as in the fast-walking group. (See Figure 4-3.) What this means is that if you are exercising to improve your level of fitness, you will have to earn your minimum weekly calorie expenditure (not less than 700 and not more than 2,000) with a certain degree of intensity. But if your only reason for starting an exercise program is to ward off diseases caused by inactivity, you can burn your calories in as leisurely a manner as you like.

Fortunately, this study also shows us that substantial improvements in cardiorespiratory fitness can occur with even moderate physical activities such as brisk walking. Still, you might be looking at this and think-

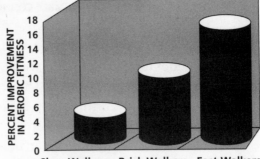

Figure 4-2.
Effect of walking speed on aerobic fitness. The findings of a
six-month study conducted by Neil and his colleagues are
shown in the above figure. Aerobic fitness was found to
increase in direct proportion to the speed at which the study
participants walked during exercise training—the faster or
more intensely they walked, the greater their improvement
in aerobic fitness. (Adapted from J. J. Duncan et al.,
"Women Walking for Health and Fitness: How Much Is
Enough?" *Journal of the American Medical Association,*
1991, 266:3295–3299.)

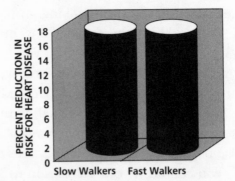

Figure 4-3.
Effect of walking speed on health. The findings of a
six-month study conducted by Neil and his colleagues are
shown in the above figure. The risk for coronary heart
disease was found to decrease to a similar degree no matter
how fast the study participants walked. (Adapted from J. J.
Duncan et al., "Women Walking for Health and Fitness: How
Much Is Enough?" *Journal of the American Medical
Association,* 1991, 266:3295–3299.)

ing, "OK, Jimmy, but I can see that in order to get the *most* cardiorespiratory fitness benefit, I have to exercise harder (more intensely)." Again, the only people who need to exercise at a very strenuous level are those athletes training for competition. And although high-intensity workouts have the advantage of accomplishing your target energy expenditure in less time, they are also associated with a much higher risk factor. Who needs it? You can raise your fitness level, improve your looks, and do wonders for your health with moderate-intensity exercise. Besides, most people don't enjoy high-intensity exercise programs and are less likely to stick to them.

If you were going to put the concept of FIT into equation form, it would look something like this:

**FREQUENCY + INTENSITY + TIME =
CALORIC ENERGY EXPENDITURE**

Think of it as you would any other addition equation. It doesn't take a math whiz to figure out that the sum of the numbers on the left, must equal the number on the right. We know that $3 + 3 + 3 = 9$. But that isn't the only way to get that total. If you changed one of the 3s to a 1, you'd have to adjust the other numbers on the left in order to get the same total: $1 + 3 + 5 = 9$. If you changed two of the numbers on the left: $2 + 2 + 5 = 9$, you'd still have to make adjustments to get to the right total. In your FIT equation, the right total is the number of calories you want to burn each week, somewhere between 700 (the low end) and 2,000 (the high end).

OK, let's go over what we know so far. We know that we have a certain amount of calories we want to burn per week during exercise and we know that we want to do so at a light- or moderate-intensity level. Good. But how in the heck are we supposed to know (a) how many calories we've burned and (b) if we've reached or gone past the right intensity level?

Intensity Level Excellent questions. Let's take the intensity question first. Until now, the most commonly recommended way to measure exercise intensity was by use of the heart rate. This method is based on the principle that there is a direct relationship between the intensity at which you exercise and your heart rate. As the intensity increases, so does the heart rate. If you exercise at an intensity that raises your heart rate to between 60 and 85 percent of your maximal heart rate, you'll be exercising at an optimal intensity for health-related fitness. In order to use this method, you would, of course, need to know what your maximal heart rate is. The most common way of determining this is to make use of an old formula: 220 − your age = your maximal heart rate. Although this formula has been used for a long time, I don't particularly care for it. My main problem with it is its lack of accuracy. Since two people of the exact same age will often have widely different maximal heart rates, the formula doesn't always work.

The only way you can accurately determine your maximal heart rate is to have your doctor measure it as part of a treadmill or cycle stress test. Even then, to make use of the information you have to figure out how to take your pulse. Trust me, unless you have someone to teach you, taking your own pulse can be a pain. I never check my heart rate, and the good doctor tells me it is only really necessary for people who have heart disease or some other chronic disease that could be worsened by inappropriate exercise.

Perceived Level of Exertion What I do, what my mother and grandmother taught me to do over thirty years ago, is *listen to my body.* In more scientific terms (I have to say it this way to make Neil happy), I monitor my *perceived level of exertion.* In other words, I keep track of how hard the exercise I'm doing feels to me.

Although it has taken me a long time to turn these feelings into a sixth sense, you won't need any time to understand what I mean. You can start monitoring your perceived level of exertion in your *next* workout. Neil has shown me a very simple, easy-to-use method of assessing our efforts that I know you will find invaluable. In fact, the only fault I can find with it is its name. This method, used by scientists and physicians all over the world, involves the use of a chart called the Borg Scale of Perceived Exertion. Neil assures me that it is not named after my longtime rival Bjorn Borg, but rather its originator, Swedish exercise physiologist Dr. Gunnar Borg. (So I guess the name stays.)

The Borg Scale helps you to judge the intensity of your workout based on your overall at-the-moment perception of how hard the exercise feels to you. It's so simple that it's brilliant. This "rating of perceived exertion,'' or RPE, is determined by the use of a scale with numbers from 6 to 20 (Figure 4-4). As you can see, next to every odd number on the scale is a description or evaluation of how the exercise feels to you. They begin at 7, which is very, very light (or easy) and continue up to 19, which is very, very hard.

When you work out, read the evaluations and then choose the number that corresponds, in your best judgment, to how difficult the exercise feels to you. In using the scale, don't concern yourself with any one reaction to your workout, such as shortness of breath or leg fatigue, but, try instead to concentrate on your overall feeling of exertion. Just be as honest as possible without underestimating or overestimating your efforts. For example, if you weren't exerting yourself in the slightest, you'd probably choose number 6 or 7. On the other hand, if you exercised to the point of exhaustion, where you couldn't take another step without collapsing (as I did during my match against Chang in the '91 French Open), you would probably pick number 20.

An RPE of 12 or 13 is the ideal range for most adults who exercise for health-related fitness. It isn't difficult or tiring enough to be unpleasant or dangerous, yet it is challenging enough to ensure that you get the most benefit from your effort. Those of you who are just starting an exercise program will gradually build up to this level. If you exercise regularly at an RPE of 12 or 13, you will successfully get down to the weight you want and be able to maintain it while also improving your fitness level and reducing your risk of disease at the same time. Even for those of you who enjoy a tough

BORG SCALE OF PERCEIVED EXERTION

	6	
	7	Very, very light
	8	
Very light	9	
	10	
	11	Fairly light
	12	
Somewhat hard	13	
	14	
	15	Hard
	16	
Very hard	17	
	18	
	19	Very, very hard
	20	

Figure 4-4.
The Borg Scale of Perceived Exertion. (From G. A. V. Borg,
"Psychophysical Bases of Perceived Exertion," *Medicine and
Science in Sports and Exercise,* 1982, 14:377–381.)

workout, there is no reason to exercise above an RPE
of 15, the number at which your perceived level of
exertion is described as "hard."

The Borg Scale figures prominently throughout the
rest of the book and in my workout programs. You
should familiarize yourself with it before you start your
exercise, keep it in mind while you are exercising, and
check it out again immediately after you have finished
exercising. You might want to make a photocopy of
the scale and keep it in your program diary, your
locker at the gym, or someplace easy to get to after

your workout. Within a few weeks, you'll know the scale by heart and, just like me, will be able to feel your own level of perceived exertion. In fact, for the purpose of my workout programs, all you really need to know is whether you're exercising below a 12, at a 12 or 13, or above a 13. Figure 4-5 will help you decide the level at which you are exerting yourself.

Calories Burned Knowing how intensely you exercise is very important, but it doesn't account for everything in your workout. You still don't know how to be sure that you burn between 700 and 2,000 calories per week. I've told you that working out for 15 to 60 minutes a day 3 to 5 days per week should be sufficient. Does that mean that if you exercise 3 days for 15 minutes a pop you will burn 700 calories and if you exercise 5 days at 60 minutes a shot you will burn 2,000 calories? No, not necessarily. The truth is that in order to know the number of calories you're burning, you have to take more into consideration than how long or often you work out. You must also consider the specific type of aerobic exercise and the intensity at which you work out. For example, five 40-minute workouts in a week could result in your burning 2,000 calories if you were working out at a moderate level of intensity (12 or 13 on the Borg Scale) and if you were doing certain aerobic activities. On the other hand, if the intensity was low and you chose different, less effective aerobic exercises, your five 40-minute workouts might not even burn the minimum 700 calories. That's a pretty big margin of error to deal with. How do you know for

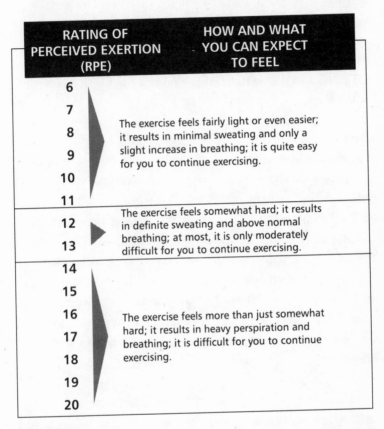

RATING OF PERCEIVED EXERTION (RPE)	HOW AND WHAT YOU CAN EXPECT TO FEEL
6	
7	
8	The exercise feels fairly light or even easier; it results in minimal sweating and only a slight increase in breathing; it is quite easy for you to continue exercising.
9	
10	
11	
12	The exercise feels somewhat hard; it results in definite sweating and above normal breathing; at most, it is only moderately difficult for you to continue exercising.
13	
14	
15	
16	The exercise feels more than just somewhat hard; it results in heavy perspiration and breathing; it is difficult for you to continue exercising.
17	
18	
19	
20	

Figure 4-5.
The Borg Scale: How and what you can expect to feel during aerobic exercise. When using my aerobic workouts, all you really need to know is whether you are exercising below a 12 on the Borg Scale, at a 12 or 13, or above a 13. This figure shows you how and what you can expect to feel at these three different levels of perceived exertion.

sure the number of calories you burn per week? This question can be answered easily once you know the Connors Count. (Now *that's* a name!)

PUTTING IT ALL TOGETHER WITH THE CONNORS COUNT

The Connors Count is a point system that incorporates everything I've discussed so far into an easy and effective way to know exactly how much exercise is enough for you. Here's how it works. Your aim is to burn 700 to 2,000 calories per week, right? Using the Connors Count, one point represents 20 calories (1 = 20). Therefore, in order to achieve the recommended score, you need to earn between 35 (35 × 20 = 700 calories) and 100 (100 × 20 = 2,000) points each week with your exercise program. To find out how many points you earn during an aerobic workout, all you need to know is:

1. the type of exercise you've performed
2. the average RPE during the workout
3. how long the workout lasted

Once you have the above information, turn to pages 192–209, where I already have the points calculated for you. After you find the points earned from your workout, it is a simple matter of adding up the points from each one. You will then know exactly how many points you've earned—or what your score is—for the week. It's that easy. Without going into a medical facility to be monitored by machines and without the time-consuming chore of making measurements such as your exact speed and distance, this is the most accurate way of judging the effectiveness of your exercise. The Connors Count is user-friendly and uncomplicated, yet it still eliminates the guesswork. (If you're wondering why you don't have to take your weight into consideration in the Connors Count, the answer is simple. Although the number of calories you burn during weight-bearing activities like walking and jogging is somewhat affected by how much you weigh, the outcome on your health and fitness probably won't be much different. The American Heart Association does not take weight into account in their recommendations for weekly energy expenditure, nor do some key studies. Because of this, Neil and I decided not to burden you with weighing yourself every time you use the Connors Count.)

One of the nicest benefits of using the Borg Scale along with the Connors Count is its ability to let you evaluate how hard you are working relative to your own capability. What I mean is this. Let's say you are a beginner when it comes to regular exercise. If you and I were to go out for a 20-minute jog together, chances are you would feel a lot more tired during that workout than I would. On the Borg Scale, I might decide that a 9 most closely represented my perceived level of exertion, while you might decide that a 13 was more accurate for how you felt. Because you are working at a higher intensity level, you would get more points in the Connors Count than I would. And rightfully so. Many of the benefits of regular exercise, especially improvements in your level of fitness, depend on how hard you work out *relative to your current fitness level*. As a result, it takes less exercise for an unfit person to improve their aerobic fitness level than for a fit person to improve their fitness level. (You know, a few years from now I think I'll lay that on some young boomer who leaves me exhausted and sweating on the court after a five-hour match. As he's trotting off into the crowd, maybe I can say something like "Hey pal, you might have had more points on the scoreboard, but I racked up more Connors Count points in the first three hours than you did all day!") The Borg Scale and the Connors Count, used together, make things fair— no matter what level of fitness you're at right now.

These two measurement tools will help you to progress gradually in the amount and intensity of your exercise until you reach your desired energy expenditure (burned calorie) goal. For example, as you become accustomed to jogging in 20-minute intervals (or whatever exercise you choose), it will no longer be such an effort. Your RPE may fall below a 12 even though you're jogging at the same pace. In order to keep earning the same amount of points in the Connors Count, you'll either have to (a) increase the intensity of your workout (jog faster), (b) keep the same intensity but jog for a longer period of time, or (c) keep the same intensity and time period but jog an extra day that week. It all comes back to the FIT equation I discussed earlier.

After about four months, you will begin to notice a plateau or stabilizing in your aerobic fitness level. This is normal. From here on you don't have to increase the time or the intensity of your workouts. If you keep your workouts the same, you'll maintain your fitness level and slow down its decline as you age. You certainly don't have to keep going faster and harder forever.

MUSCULAR STRENGTH AND STRETCHING EXERCISES

In some ways, it's much easier to talk about how much muscle strengthening and stretching you need in order to optimize your health-related fitness. I say "in some ways" because although I know how to build strength, I don't incorporate strength training into my own weekly routine. The reason I don't is that I need to maintain a delicate balance between my various muscle groups in order to achieve my best results on the tennis court. Right now I get all the strength training I need from the intensity with which I hold the racquet, combined with the force with which I hit the ball in my serve, forehand, and two-handed backhand shots. The same principle applies for my not having to include any stretching exercises into my workout program. I get all the benefits of a regular flexibility routine from swinging the racquet and reaching for the ball when I play tennis. However, I believe that both these types of exercise are important to do on a regular basis and will use them in a manner similar to the way you do after I quit playing competitive tennis.

From a health standpoint, too little research has been done to know the exact amounts of muscle strength and flexibility exercise needed to help prevent chronic diseases related to inactivity. Still, from a fitness standpoint these exercises are quite valuable, so we should talk about them. How important they are to you depends largely on the nature of your lifestyle.

Muscular strength can be developed by using either of two types of resistance exercises: *isometric* resistance exercises and/or *dynamic* resistance exercises. Isometric resistance exercises involve the tensing (or contracting) of one set of muscles against the other or against an immovable object.

For example, when you place the palms of your hands together and push, or grip the sides of the chair you're sitting on and pull up, and then hold these positions for a couple of seconds, you have performed isometric exercise. Little or no joint movement takes place. Like isometrics, dynamic resistance exercises also require the contraction of your muscles. But unlike isometrics, they involve movement of a joint or limb. Weight lifting is a typical dynamic muscle-strengthening exercise.

The American College of Sports Medicine recommends dynamic resistance exercise when working out for health-related fitness. As a healthy adult, you should perform an average of 8 to 10 dynamic resistance exercises involving your major muscle groups a minimum of two times per week. For each exercise you choose, you should do at least one set of 8 to 12 repetitions. Sure, if you do more than this, you may get stronger and develop larger muscles, but from a health-related fitness standpoint the gains are not that important. So once more I say, why bother? Your time is too valuable to spend a lot of effort doing something that is not going to make that much of a difference.

As in your aerobic workout, you will go to the Borg Scale to determine if the amount of weight you are using is right for you. When it comes to muscle strengthening you should strive for an RPE of 12 to 15. (See Figure 4-6.) Progression is an important principle when it comes to improving muscle strength and endurance. Therefore, when you first begin strength training, it would be to your advantage to start off with a light weight and 8 repetitions (or fewer if necessary) and build to 12 repetitions. Once that routine becomes too easy for you, you should increase the weight and go back to 8 repetitions and build to 12 as before. After a few months of increasing this progression, your strength gains will start to plateau or stabilize. When you reach this point your goal should be maintenance—to preserve the strength you've worked so hard to develop.

It doesn't matter whether you perform your muscle-strengthening exercises before, after, or in the middle of your aerobic workout. What does matter is that you be sure to leave at least 48 hours between your strength-training exercises when they involve the same muscle group. In other words, don't work on strengthening the same muscle group two days in a row. If you want to work out with weights Monday and Tuesday, for example, you would work on your arms on Monday and your legs on Tuesday.

Muscle-strengthening exercises, like the ones outlined in my programs later in the book, can be performed at home with the use of hand-held weights (dumbbells). They can also be performed with free weights or dynamic resistance exercise machines

RATING OF PERCEIVED EXERTION (RPE)	HOW AND WHAT YOU CAN EXPECT TO FEEL
6 7 8 9 10 11	The weight or resistance feels fairly light to you; it is fairly easy for you to complete all of your repetitions.
12 13 14 15	The weight or resistance feels somewhat heavy or even heavy to you; it is somewhat hard or difficult for you to complete all of your repetitions.
16 17 18 19 20	The weight or resistance feels very heavy to you; it is extremely hard if not impossible for you to complete all of your repetitions.

Figure 4-6.
The Borg Scale: How and What You Can Expect to Feel During Strength Training. The Borg Scale can help you determine if the amount of weight or the resistance you are using is right for you. Ideally, you should rate your exertion at a 12 to 15 during each set of 8 to 12 repetitions of an exercise. This figure shows you how and what you can expect to feel at three different levels of perceived exertion.

found in gyms. It is very important that you get someone qualified to carefully instruct you in the correct
way to use free weights and these machines.

The American College of Sports Medicine (you probably think I graduated from there, don't you?) does not
have similar guidelines for stretching. Until further
studies are made available, I recommend that when it
comes to reducing the risk of injuring yourself during
your workouts, you should place more emphasis on
warming up correctly than on performing specific
stretching exercises. I don't walk out on the court and
expect to serve aces or hit winners immediately. (It
takes a good 3 minutes before that happens.) I start off
slowly and gently take my joints through their range of
motion during my warm-up period on the court. In
much the same way you should take at least 3 minutes
to increase gradually the intensity of your aerobic
workout until you reach your desired level. For example, walk briskly before jogging or begin jogging at a
slower pace. If you cycle, pedal slower or apply less
resistance during the first few minutes. When doing
muscle-strengthening exercises, use a lighter weight or
less resistance for your first set of each different exercise. If in addition to warming up you like to perform
actual stretching exercises, try 2 or 3 gentle repetitions
of the ones described in the photo insert of my workout
programs.

When performing stretching exercises, you should
be aware that they are best done after at least 5 minutes
of mild aerobic exercise. Why? Because the exercise
raises the temperature of the tissues surrounding your

joints, making them more supple and less prone to injury. This is why, in order to get the greatest improvements in long-term flexibility, your stretching exercises should be done *after*—rather than *before*—your aerobic workout. And unless you regularly participate in physical activities such as tennis that will provide you with the flexibility training you need, I do encourage you to include the stretching exercises shown in Chapter 7 at the end of each of your aerobic workouts.

It is important for you to remember that when doing stretching exercises you should gently stretch to the point of tension and hold the position for about 8 to 12 seconds. Don't stretch to the point of pain. Avoid bouncing, as it could result in injury. I can tell you this from experience. Once, while waiting through a rain delay at a tournament, I was having a case of the butterflies (after all these years, I still get those damn butterflies). I had already warmed up and didn't want to lose the feeling before the match started again. To keep myself busy I started to move my chest from side to side, thinking the stretch would do me good. I guess I was a little rough, because the next thing I felt was the muscles in my chest tearing. The pain was excruciating and, needless to say, I didn't win the match. The point is that although stretching may seem like an easy thing to do, it should be treated with the same amount of respect as any other form of exercise. Please, learn from my mistake. I don't want you to get hurt.

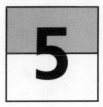

Don't Work Your Lifestyle— Make Your Lifestyle Work

PROBABLY THE MOST frequently used excuse for not exercising regularly is "I don't have time." True, regular exercise *does* require a certain amount of commitment. But let's be honest. Whenever we really want to do something, we *find* the time, somewhere. There's an old saying that goes: "If you want to get something done, give it to a busy person to do." For whatever reason, a busy person finds time to do everything. I know that even for me, on those few days a year when I have only a couple of things on my schedule, the temptation to procrastinate is strong. I figure I have all day to get them done. Pretty soon, the end of the day is here, and unless I forced myself to take action, nothing happened.

If you perceive that lack of time is your reason for not exercising, I think I can help. Now that you understand the Connors Count, I'll show you how to put it to use for yourself in another way. The idea of working a regular exercise program into your lifestyle doesn't have to be an overwhelming concept. The trick is to make your lifestyle work for you as best as you can right now. Then you'll need to add less formal exercise training to your schedule in order to score the desired 35 to 100 points each week.

Within this system, you can actually score points for almost every physical activity you do. Not just your regular workouts, but *everything*. Do you walk to work? Could you? That counts. Walk your dog? That counts too. Have to climb three flights of stairs to your apartment? Give yourself some points. Hell, if you jogged up and down those steps, you'd get even more! You see, it's very possible you're *already* racking up more points in a week than you think, just by doing the things you have to do to get by. When you add up all those little points, the time you actually have to spend on a scheduled aerobic workout could be significantly less than you anticipated. The Connors Count was developed for one purpose—to make your life easier.

What you need to remember is it's not only what you do, but also how you do it. In other words, you need to take into account what kind of activity you did, how long you did it, and your perceived exertion on the Borg Scale. With that information in hand, simply turn to the charts on pages 192–209, note the Connors Count score, and start keeping score on a daily basis. For example, let's say you walk your dog Pluto every morning from 7:00 to 7:30. I can't give you the exact number of points you'd receive for that without knowing how you rated your exertion level, but you would score some points. Chances are, you could walk Pluto in the evening as well. If you walked faster, your effort would be greater and you'd score more points. Maybe you could encourage Pluto to break into a slow trot on the way home and earn yet even more points.

You don't always have to interrupt your normal schedule to get exercise. Be a little creative and you could accumulate enough points right now to improve your health without actually starting the kind of formal exercise program I'll show you in Chapter 7. In order to get and stay fitter than you are right now, you will probably have to incorporate a few extra exercise sessions into your regular weekly schedule. But by putting a little more elbow grease into the effort with which you perform your everyday activities you could literally cut that time in half.

Here are a few suggestions that may give you some ideas on how to make your current lifestyle work better to benefit your body, your appearance, and your health:

1. Walk to work. If that isn't possible, drive or ride part of the way and walk or ride a bike the rest of the distance.

2. Take a walk during break periods or at lunch.

3. Climb the stairs instead of using an elevator or escalator. If you're going to a high floor in a building, let's say 24, take the elevator up to floor 14 and walk the rest of the way.

4. When at a mall, the movies, a restaurant, or an airport, park your car farther away from the entrance than you normally would. (Be careful to find a spot that is well lit so that you're not walking around in the dark late at night.)

5. Say "Yes" when your kids or grandchildren ask you to go to the park or come out and play with them.

6. Mow your own lawn and/or work outside in the garden.

I hope these suggestions will give you an idea of what I mean. There are a lot of different ways to score points with the Connors Count. To make it fun for yourself, try comparing the number of points you get in a week with what a couple of your friends score. Then before starting one of the two programs in this book, try to come up with easy ways of earning more points without changing your routine. I think it's interesting to know how many points I can score without even going for the big effort. I have a feeling you'll be surprised too.

Another way I've found of getting more points for the week is making use of what I call "downtime." Downtime includes that time lost while standing in line or waiting for the commercials on television to end. You know what I mean, the kinds of nonactivities that can drive you crazy, but they are all in a day's work. They can't be avoided, so why not make the most of them?

Whenever I have to wait in line for more than a few minutes for anything, I get impatient. I do it, but I always feel like I'm wasting time. What I do to compensate is keep moving. If I can jog in place, or walk around while I wait, the time doesn't seem so misspent. My movements may not help the line move any faster, but I don't lose my cool. And I don't know about you, but except for a couple of those really clever Nuprin, Power-stick, and Pepsi commercials, I can't stand having a television program interrupted by ads. But once again, I can't do anything about it, so I try to make the most of the moment. Sometimes I'll jump rope during those few minutes. Other times I'll race one of the kids to the mailbox or run outside and shoot a couple of baskets with Brett. These are my ways of turning downtime into uptime.

Of course, sometimes I just need to relax and do nothing, which can also be productive. I'll talk about this more in Chapter 9, but I wanted you to know that I am not trying to think of a way to exercise during every waking moment. Relaxation is one of the joys in life and I do it regularly. Everyone should. These little tricks are for those times when you'd rather be exercising but can't.

After you figure out how many points you're already scoring in the Connors Count and how many more you could easily earn without changing your routine, it will be time to consider what type of exercise you'll want to fit into your lifestyle in order to make up the difference between what you already have and what you still need to reach those 35 to 100 points.

I have found that the variety in my program is what keeps it fresh and exciting. I don't have a long attention span and I tend to get bored fast in my training. Because every game is different, I don't have that problem when playing tennis. I never know where the ball is going to come from and that excitement keeps the sport stimulating for me. But my workout programs involve different kinds of exercise, as you'll see. I like to mix it up. Today, there are so many types of exercise available, it is unlikely that you won't find something you enjoy. I have set up my programs in a way that leaves you choices. For every exercise I do I've listed options that you can use to make substitutions that will give you a similar number of points. You can either follow my programs exactly as they are written or pick the exercise of your choice. If you decide to make a substitution, you'll still be doing the Jimmy Connors Workout, but you'll have tailored it to fit your needs.

The most variety seems to be available in aerobic exercise. Let's talk about some of the most popular forms of aerobic exercise and their potential benefits. Remember, the ideal exercise has four basic characteristics:

1. It's pleasant to do. An exercise you enjoy is one you're more likely to stick with.

2. It should be practical to do and fit your lifestyle. You'll want to find something you can do all year.

3. It should use large muscle groups. The larger the muscle groups involved in your exercise effort, the greater the amount of oxygen you'll be using and the greater the amount of calories you'll burn. (More points.)

4. It should not impose excessive stress on your joints that could result in injury.

Walking and Jogging I enjoy jogging around my property and through the hills surrounding my home. I like being outside and breathing fresh air. Spending so much time in California makes it easy for me to do this much of the year. Jogging up and down the hills not only improves my endurance but strengthens my legs, both of which come in handy during a five-set match.

Before you include jogging of any kind in your exercise routine, start off with a walking program and then a walk-jog program. It took me years to build up to the level of fitness that I'm at today.

Jogging in the hills is especially strenuous and should be limited to once a week, even for those who are in great shape. If you eventually incorporate hill jogging into your program, be sure to stick to the perceived exertion (RPE) guidelines discussed in Chapter 4. In fact, unless you are particularly gung ho on it, you don't even have to jog in order to optimize your health-related fitness. Walking is just as effective. Like jogging, it's a simple exercise requiring no special skill, setting, or equipment other than a good pair of walking shoes. Its major advantage over jogging, especially for those of you who are just beginning to exercise, is that it's far less stressful on your joints. During jogging, your feet strike the ground with a force that is usually equal to three or four times your body weight. This force is transmitted to your ankles, knees, and hips and could cause injury if overdone. In contrast, walking only exerts a force of one and a half times your weight on these joints.

Neil tells me that walking fast burns nearly as many calories as jogging slowly. So you can increase your cardiorespiratory fitness level without the risk of injury. Walking with light hand weights (1 to 3 pounds) is another way to up your energy expenditure without resorting to jogging, as long as you swing your arms more vigorously than usual. Sometimes, however, these exaggerated movements can disrupt your normal biomechanics and make you *more* prone to injury. This is why I would rather recommend walking faster or farther to make up the extra points. In bad weather, walking or jogging on a treadmill is an alternative to exercising outdoors. Most treadmills have an incline setting to simulate hills. And, just for the record, walking uphill on a treadmill burns almost 30 percent more calories for a given rating of perceived exertion than walking on a level surface. This kind of walking is an excellent form of aerobic exercise.

Jumping Rope My grandfather was a boxer and included jumping rope as part of his regular exercise routine. He encouraged me to jump rope along with him in my early teens and I've been doing it ever since. It is a terrific form of aerobic exercise and in the process improves quickness, coordination, agility, rhythm, and timing. Not only that, but jumping rope is inexpensive, is portable, and doesn't require special facilities or weather conditions.

As with any other form of strenuous exercise, you must start gradually and build up as your fitness level improves. If you haven't exercised in a long time, introduce jumping rope after about 8 to 12 weeks of lower-intensity aerobic exercise, such as fast walking or slow jogging. Jumping rope at an average rate (approximately 130 jumps per minute) is about as strenuous as jogging a 9- or 10-minute mile.

For beginners, it is even more strenuous than that and can't be done for more than a couple of minutes at a time. That's why in one of my programs I suggest alternating brief periods of jumping rope with brief periods of marching in place.

If you decide to try jumping rope, and I highly recommend it for those of you who have never had problems with your joints, make sure you get the right rope for you. The length is very important, so don't buy the kind that stretches when you pull on it. The end of the handles should just reach your armpits when you stand on the middle of the rope. To reduce your risk of injury, wear aerobic or cross-training shoes. They have extra cushioning at the ball of the foot, which is where you land. Try to avoid jumping on very hard surfaces such as concrete and tile. If you feel you're working too hard, march in place or move on to a less strenuous exercise, like walking. What I do is jump for 3 minutes, then rest for 1 minute. Be aware that attempting to jump slower will not expend less energy because when you jump slower, you have to jump higher to keep time with the turning rope. Finally, jumping rope is best done in conjunction with other forms of exercise rather than as your only form of aerobic activity. It should also be limited to no more than 3 sessions per week. Jumping rope every day will increase your risk of shin splints and calf injuries.

Stair Climbing This is another one of my favorite forms of exercise. I like it because it enables me to use large muscle groups in my back, buttocks, and legs at the same time. Although I have a stair-climbing machine in my home, this form of aerobic activity is one I can do anywhere. On the road, I will often climb up and down stairs in my hotel to get the same workout benefits. Using the stairs at work, at shopping malls, or at home can be done easily without incurring the cost of a machine. As with anything else, stair climbing presents its own risk of injury when not done in moderation. It has been estimated that the stress stair climbing places on the knee joint is about the same as lifting four to six times your body weight. Again, this exercise should be limited to no more than 3 sessions each week. If you are just beginning an exercise program, wait until you've been working out for at least 8 to 12 weeks before adding it to your routine.

Cycling Stationary and outdoor cycling are more popular than ever. Stationary cycling machines are great because they allow you the freedom to do other things, like read or watch TV while you exercise. They also eliminate the excuse of not being able to work out because of bad weather. A variety of stationary bikes are available, and some are even made to work your arms and upper body as well as your legs. These dual-action bikes are my favorite because they allow me to burn more calories than the others. Stationary cycling puts less stress on the joints than jogging, jumping rope, and stair climbing, so it can be incorporated into your program right away. To reduce any risk of stress on the knee, be sure to set the seat height to where your knee joint is almost (but not completely) straight while pedaling. Some people complain about getting sore buttocks while riding. To eliminate this rather touchy problem, lift up off the seat for a few seconds and then reposition yourself. You can also buy cushioned seats in many sporting goods shops.

Although stationary cycling has its advantages, for some people there is still nothing like going for a ride outdoors. I happen to be one of those people. I like going out for long rides with the family because it gives us a chance to be together without interruptions. Of course, cycling outside presents its own set of drawbacks. If you ride in traffic, there can be lots of starts and stops, which decrease your energy expenditure and therefore the aerobic benefit. The danger of falling is another consideration. For this reason, it is always a good idea to wear a protective helmet. Who cares if they look a little weird? I'd much rather look funny and reduce my and my family's risk of injury than give up the helmets for the sake of vanity. Fortunately, we live out of the mainstream of traffic. City dwellers should consider packing the bikes on the car and driving to a place safe from a lot of oncoming vehicles. Then you can enjoy the fresh air and sunshine while getting the most from your workout at the same time.

Swimming As you have probably figured out by now, I love being outside. That's why swimming has always been a favorite exercise of mine. Unfortunately, I can only do it recreationally rather than as part of my program because I found that swimming gives my upper body too much of a workout. This focus on upper-body muscles conflicts with the balance I need to play my best tennis. Even so, I highly recommend it for others because it works so many large muscle groups all over the body. In addition to being an excellent aerobic workout, because swimming is a non-weight-bearing activity it provides a minimal risk of injury. The traditional way to work out in the water is swimming laps. Master's swim programs are popping up all over the country, both outdoors and indoors, and have generated a new interest in lap swimming. These programs are a great way to improve your health-related fitness level.

Another pool program that is becoming extremely popular is "aqua-aerobics." As the name implies, this is aerobic exercise done while submerged in water. It increases your strength, flexibility, and cardiorespiratory fitness all at the same time. This form of exercise is so gentle on the joints that many injured athletes can do it regularly while recovering from their injuries.

The only drawbacks to swimming are that you must, of course, find a pool or body of water to work out in and you must know how to swim. Also, those of you who are exercising for the specific purpose of losing weight may be disappointed to learn that although swimming is an excellent way to improve cardiorespiratory fitness, a recent study, according to Neil, suggests it may not be as successful in decreasing body fat as some of the other exercises I've talked about.

Aerobic Dancing I don't need to tell you how popular aerobic dancing is today. It seems as if everyone is doing it. The idea is that if you're dancing, you're hav-

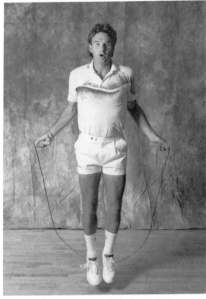

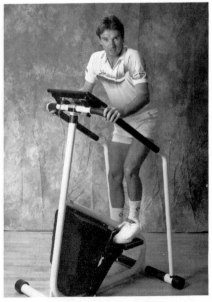

Jumping Rope. This is a terrific form of aerobic exercise and definitely one of my favorites.

Stair Climbing. Stair climbing enables you to expend large amounts of energy. It is another one of my favorite forms of aerobic exercise.

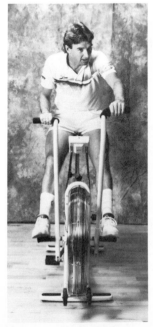

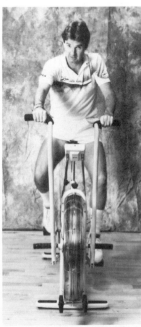

Stationary Cycling. Stationary cycling machines eliminate the excuse of not being able to work out because of bad weather. A variety of excellent cycles are available. Some dual-action bikes enable you to use your arms and legs at the same time (as I am on the right). Alternatively, you can use your legs or (as I'm doing on the left) your arms alone, should you wish to.

The Importance of Correct Technique During Strength Training. Be sure to maintain good posture and use the correct technique when performing muscle strengthening exercises. In this photo, I am discussing correct technique with Dr. Neil Gordon.

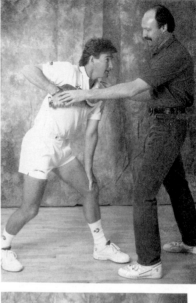

Recommended stretching exercises to improve your flexibility. Do 2 to 3 repetitions of each of these exercises at the end of your aerobic workouts. Hold each stretch for 8 to 12 seconds with no bouncing. Stretch to the point of tension, not pain.

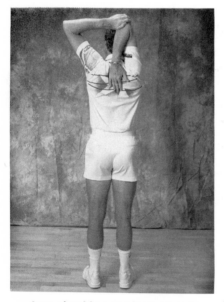

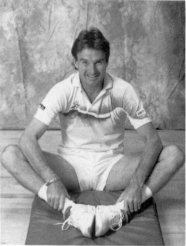

Arm, shoulder, and back stretch. Lift your right elbow toward the ceiling and place your right hand as far down your back between the shoulder blades as possible. Allow your chin to rest on your chest. If possible, using your left hand, gently pull your right elbow to the left until a stretch is felt on the back of the right arm and down the right side of the back. Hold. Repeat with the left arm.

Inner thigh stretch. Sit on the floor, place the soles of your feet together, grasp your ankles, and pull your heels in fairly close to you. Place your elbows against the inside of your knees and gently press your knees down toward the floor.

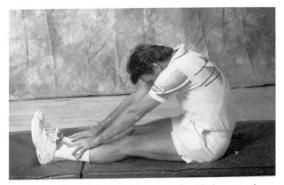

Lower back and hamstring stretch. Sitting on the floor with legs straight out in front and hands on thighs, bend forward slowly, gently reaching toward your toes. Keep head and back aligned as you move into the stretch. If necessary, you may bend your knees slightly.

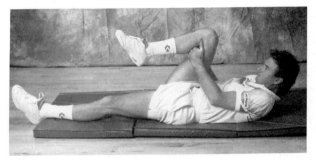

Lower back and thigh stretch. Lie flat on your back with your legs extended on the floor, then pull (grasp under rather than in front of your knees) the right knee gently up to your chest. Press your back to the floor. Hold the position and then repeat with the left knee.

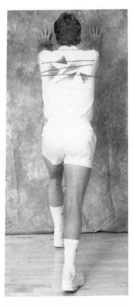

Calf stretch. Stand facing a wall, approximately three feet away. Place your palms on the wall and keep feet flat on the floor. Keep one foot in place and step forward with the other foot. Keep the back leg straight and gently bend the front knee forward toward the wall. Repeat with the opposite leg. (If you are a jogger or rope jumper, this is one exercise that is beneficial to perform before as well as after exercise—it may help reduce your risk for Achilles tendon and calf injuries.)

The Jimmy Connors Home Muscle Strengthening Program. In each of my 16-week programs you will find recommendations on how much strength training you should include in your weekly exercise regimen. If you don't have access to a gym, you can still benefit by doing the exercises shown here. When using them remember to follow the safety guidelines I outlined in the previous chapter. Of the ten exercises, nine involve the use of dumbbells. I suggest that women start out with a weight no heavier than 3 pounds if they are not used to weight training, and men with a weight no heavier than 6 pounds. When moving up to a heavier weight do so in small increments as your capacity permits. Be sure to maintain good posture throughout each exercise. Perform each exercise with controlled movements. By returning the dumbbells to the starting position slowly, in a controlled fashion, you will derive added benefit from each exercise—don't swing the dumbbells. For those of you who do have access to a gym or any of the various resistance training machines that are available, I've provided the names of some suitable exercises that could be used in place of the ones shown here (where appropriate)—please have someone who is experienced in their correct usage show you how to perform them.

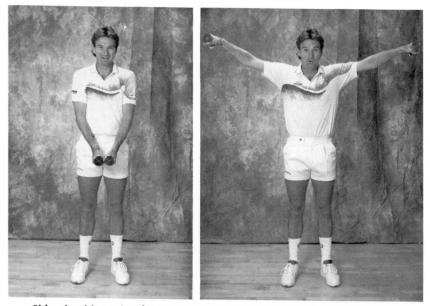

Side shoulder raise (strengthens outer portion of the shoulders). Start with arms hanging in front of thighs, elbows slightly bent, and palms facing each other. Raise both dumbbells outward simultaneously to about shoulder height, keeping elbows slightly bent. Lower dumbbells to starting position and repeat. (Suggested alternative: military press.)

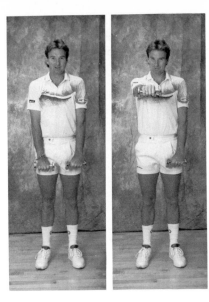

Front shoulder raise (strengthens front portion of the shoulders). Start with arms hanging in front of thighs and palms facing thighs. Raise one dumbbell straight in front of you to about shoulder height. Lower dumbbell to starting position and repeat using other arm. Alternate arms. (Suggested alternatives: military press; push-up.)

Upright row (strengthens shoulders, neck, and upper back). Start with arms hanging in front of thighs, palms facing thighs, and dumbbells touching each other. Keeping dumbbells close to the body and in contact with each other, raise them simultaneously to about chin height. Lower dumbbells to starting position and repeat. (Suggested alternatives: upright row using barbell; pull-up; lat pull-down.)

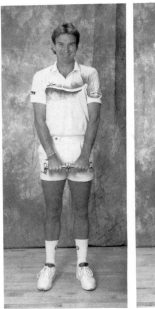
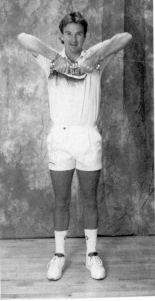

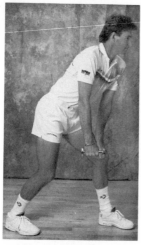
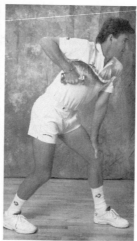

One-arm row (strengthens upper back and shoulders). Place one foot about a step in front of the other, bend the front knee slightly, lean forward, and rest your free hand, palm down, on the knee of your front leg. Let the arm holding the dumbbell hang straight at your side. Raise the dumbbell up toward your armpit. Lower dumbbell to starting position and repeat. After completing the desired number of repetitions, repeat with the other arm. (Suggested alternatives: seated row; lat pull-down; pull-up.)

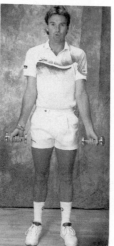
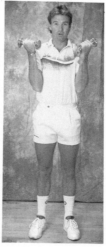

Biceps curl (strengthening of biceps, or front of the upper arm). Start with arms hanging at sides and palms facing away from your body. Keeping the elbows close to your sides, curl both dumbbells upward to the shoulders. Lower and repeat. (Suggested alternatives: barbell or machine bicep curls.)

Triceps extension (strengthening of the triceps, or back of the upper arm). Place one foot about a step in front of the other, bend the front knee slightly, lean forward, and rest your free hand, palm down, on the knee of your front leg. Place the hand holding the dumbbell against your hip (palm of hand facing the hip). Keeping the elbow still, straighten the arm fully behind you. Then bend your elbow, returning the dumbbell to your hip, and repeat. After completing the desired number of repetitions, repeat with the other arm. (Suggested alternatives: triceps push-down; dips; push-up.)

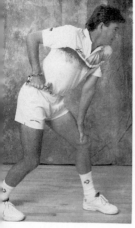
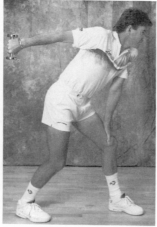

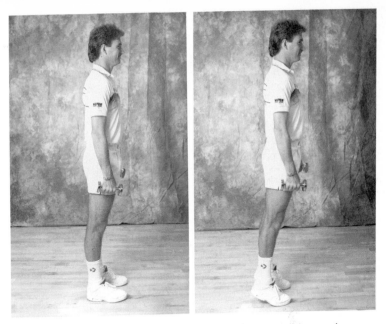

Calf raises (strengthening of the calf muscles). Start with arms hanging at sides, dumbbells in hands, and feet slightly apart. Rise onto the balls of both feet without bending the knees. Lower heels to the floor and repeat. (Suggested alternatives: standing calf raise machine; seated calf raises.)

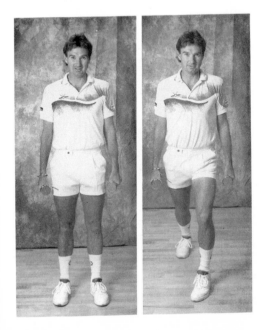

Lunges (strengthening of thigh muscles, buttocks). Start with arms hanging at sides, dumbbells in hands, and feet apart. Take a step forward with one foot and bend the front knee. Step back to starting position and repeat with opposite leg. Keep your back straight throughout the exercise. (Suggested alternatives: leg press; squats; knee extension; knee curl.)

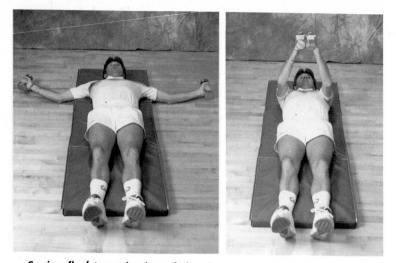

Supine fly (strengthening of the chest muscles). Lie faceup on the floor with knees straight or bent, whichever is more comfortable. With dumbbells in your hands, place your arms on the floor at right angles to your body. With elbows slightly bent, raise both dumbbells above your chest to meet in the center. Lower dumbbells out to the side and repeat. (Suggested alternatives: bench press; seated machine fly; push-up.)

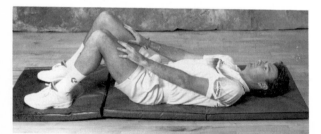

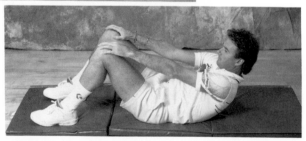

Sit-ups (strengthening of the abdominal muscles). Lie faceup on the floor with knees bent at a 90-degree angle and the palms of your hands resting on your thighs. Lift your shoulders off the floor and slide your fingers up toward your knees. Return to the starting position and repeat.

ing fun. You can do it without a partner. You can do it at home by yourself along with a video or in a class with other people. Aerobic dancing is not something I do personally because I get all the cardiorespiratory exercise I need from my other workouts. Still, there are enough different kinds of classes and videos available to make this kind of workout interesting and effective too. Make sure you wear a shoe that gives you the kind of support you need for the type of dancing you're doing. I think it's a good idea to take a class or two if you're just starting an exercise program, even if you prefer to dance along with a video at home after that. You'll want to make sure you're doing the moves correctly to avoid getting hurt. Remember to note your RPE and slow down when you feel uncomfortable.

Recreational Sports As you know, I am a big fan of recreational sports. Besides tennis, I love to shoot baskets with Brett and some of my buddies, as well as kick a soccer ball around. I believe in the camaraderie of organized sports. I think they increase sportsmanship and teach the value of being a team player. If you don't belong to a sports team of any kind, you might want to consider starting one with some of your friends. Whether it involves softball, round-robin tennis, basketball, volleyball, or anything else, meeting for a game a couple of times a week can give you a good number of Connors Count points and let you hang out with your friends while you're at it.

I could go on forever about the different kinds of aerobic exercise. The point is, there are a lot of them.

I know that with a little imagination and experimentation, you'll be able to find a few that appeal to you. It is important to at least try a variety of exercises before settling into a regular program. If you try them and decide they're not for you, that's one thing. But if you only do one exercise all the time, you may miss something you enjoy more or that works better for you. And if you find activities that bring you pleasure, you'll have a hell of a lot more fun and end up with a program that doesn't disappoint you.

When you try to work your lifestyle around exercise, the effort is too great—for anyone. That's why I only do the kinds of exercise I enjoy. Believe me when I tell you that I've tried a lot of things I didn't like and they are not in my personal routine. That doesn't mean they're no good and they shouldn't be in yours. You have to find the exercises that make you feel as good as mine make me feel. Beyond that, give yourself credit for where you are right now and the fact that you're willing to make a change for the better. Figure out the amount of Connors Count points you've earned with your everyday activities before you take on the responsibility of adding more. You may not need to add as many as you think. This is what I call making your lifestyle work. It is the core of my philosophy and why I believe my life has been a success. It will also give you the power to meet your own goals. I can talk all day long about which exercises are right for me. But if they don't fit into your lifestyle or you don't find them enjoyable, why should you care? Remember, my friends, the only *good* exercise is the kind you *do*.

THE

JIMMY

CONNORS

WORKOUT

PROGRAM—

FEATURING THE
CONNORS COUNT

PART TWO

6

Practicing Safe Exercise

BY NOW YOU'RE probably thinking, "Hey, Jimmy, quit talking about your program and give it to me already!" Well, it's coming in the next chapter—I promise. But before you begin, there are some medical guidelines you should be aware of in order to ensure your safety and get the most out of the Jimmy Connors Workout. Although you are *much* more likely to place your health in jeopardy by *not* allowing your body to move regularly, I wouldn't be doing either of us any favors if I sent you out there without at least discussing what you can do to make the experience as safe and pleasant as possible.

For this, I'm turning the floor over to the good doctor, Neil Gordon. This is his thing and I believe he

knows best. You should know that I have been following these guidelines more closely now that I've turned
40, and I recommend that they be taken seriously by
everyone, especially those of us over 35.

SAFE EXERCISE GUIDELINES

**1. Know whether you should see a doctor
before starting your exercise program or
increasing your current level of physical activity.**

Most exercise books provide a medical disclaimer en-
couraging everyone to see a doctor before beginning
on a program of regular exercise or increasing their
current level of physical activity. For many reasons,
such as lack of time or money, or a feeling of "I know
my body better than anyone," most people don't.

I recommend that you use the following approach,
which is based on the guidelines of the American College of Sports Medicine, to determine if you need to
consult your doctor before starting either of Jimmy's
programs.

If you place a check mark next to any of the state-
ments listed below, do go ahead and see a physician,
just to be safe. Bring the program you plan to start to
your doctor so he or she will know your intentions and
can guide you accordingly. Both you and your doctor
should be aware that Jimmy's programs are not intended for those of you with chronic illnesses or other

conditions that may be worsened by unsupervised exercise.

_____ I'm a male over age 40 or a female over age 50, and intend to perform vigorous exercise (exercise that will cause me to rate my perceived exertion at a 13 or higher).

_____ I intend to participate in vigorous exercise and I have two or more of the following risk factors for coronary heart disease: high blood pressure; a blood-cholesterol level above 239 mg/dl; smoke cigarettes; diabetes; a family history of heart disease in parents or siblings under age 55.

_____ I suffer from symptoms (such as chest pain or discomfort) that may be related to a major chronic disease (such as heart disease, lung disease, stroke, diabetes, or arthritis).

_____ I have a chronic disease or a health problem that is of concern to me.

If you _did not_ place a check mark next to any of the above, complete the Physical Activity Readiness Questionnaire, or PAR-Q, on the next page to further ensure that you do not need to consult a physician before beginning one of Jimmy's workouts.

Once you've completed either one of his 16-week programs presented in the next chapter, you should reassess your need to see a doctor on a yearly basis and before increasing your exercise intensity to a level that will give you a perceived exertion rating of a 13 or higher.

If at any time you should experience any disturbing symptoms at all, don't hesitate to see a physician. You've heard it before, but it is always better to be safe than sorry where your health is concerned.

The Physical Activity Readiness Questionnaire This is a revised version of the PAR-Q. It has been designed to identify the small number of adults for whom physical activity might be inappropriate or those who should have medical advice concerning the type of exercise most suitable for them.

Common sense is your best guideline in answering these questions. Read them carefully and answer "Yes" or "No" for each question as it applies to you. If you answer "No" to all questions, you may proceed with either of Jimmy's programs with a high level of confidence provided you follow the remaining safe exercise guidelines. If you answer "Yes" to one or more questions, consult your physician.

1. Has a doctor ever said you have a heart condition?
2. Do you have chest pain (or discomfort) brought on by physical activity?
3. Have you recently developed chest pain (or discomfort) that has not been checked out by your doctor?
4. Do you often feel faint or have spells of severe dizziness?

5. Do you have a bone or joint problem, such as arthritis, that could be aggravated by the exercises discussed in this book?
6. Has a doctor ever recommended medication for your blood pressure or a heart condition?
7. Are you presently under a doctor's care for any disease or condition?
8. Are you aware, through your own experience or doctor's advice, of *any* other physical reason (including pregnancy and breast feeding) which would deter your exercising without medical supervision or specific instructions from a doctor?

2. Be thoroughly versed in the warning signs of an impending cardiac complication.

Once you've been cleared to participate in Jimmy's programs, either by the PAR-Q or by your doctor, you can lower your risk even further by remembering that although death during exercise is always unexpected, it's seldom *unheralded.*

In other words, you are very likely to have some warning signs that something is not right. Here are the most obvious bodily signs that all may not be well with your heart. Should you experience any, discuss them with your doctor before continuing with your exercise program.

• *Pain or discomfort in your chest, abdomen, back, neck, jaw, or arms.* Particularly when brought on by exercise and relieved by slowing down or stopping completely, such symptoms may be indicative of an inadequate supply of blood and oxygen to your heart muscle.

• *Nauseous sensation during or shortly after exercise.* While this can be brought on by a variety of causes, such as pushing yourself too hard, too early in the program, it can also signify a cardiac abnormality.

• *Unaccustomed shortness of breath during exercise.* Obviously, moderate or intense exercise makes you breathe harder than when you're at rest. This isn't what I'm talking about. If you ordinarily walk briskly for 30 minutes without breathlessness and all of a sudden can no longer do it, you should be concerned.

• *Dizziness or actual fainting.* This can occur even in healthy people who don't cool down adequately after their workout. Anyone who stops exercising suddenly may feel momentarily dizzy. The type of dizziness that should mainly concern you happens *during* rather than immediately following exercise. If this happens to you, see a doctor right away.

• *An irregular pulse, especially when it has been regular in previous workouts.* If you check your pulse during exercise and notice what seem to be skipped or extra heartbeats, notify your doctor. It could mean nothing serious, but it is sometimes a warning of heart problems.

3. Always warm up and cool down adequately.

Most cardiac complications associated with exercise happen at the beginning or the end of a session. Such problems can be minimized by always including a warm-up and a cool-down with each workout. As Jimmy mentioned earlier, warming up before a session may also reduce your risk for injury during exercise.

The easiest way to warm up for aerobic exercise is to simply start the activity at a low intensity and gradually increase it over a period of at least 3 minutes until you reach your desired intensity level. If you cross-train— do more than one type of aerobic activity during a single workout—there is no need to repeat this warm-up when immediately changing from one exercise to the next.

Similarly, cooling down after aerobic exercise is usually best accomplished by gradually reducing the intensity of your exercise over a period of at least 3 minutes. Don't stop exercising suddenly and stand completely motionless. Always walk it out. This will help prevent the sudden drop in blood pressure that occurs with the abrupt ending of intense physical activity.

4. Start slowly and progress gradually.

I always tell my new patients that they should end their first few exercise sessions feeling that the program is so easy that they may be wasting their time. This advice is given to everyone starting a new program, even those who go on to run marathons.

There are a couple of reasons why your entry into this new world of frequent exercise should be gradual. A slow start helps prevent injuries because it allows your muscles, bones, tendons, ligaments, and joints a chance to adapt slowly to the newfound stresses of exercise. The number one cause of injury is simply doing too much, too soon. Also, a gradual progression gives you the opportunity to adjust mentally to this new way of life. If you relax and enjoy the process of change, you'll be more likely to stick with Jimmy's programs for life.

5. Take the necessary steps to minimize your risk of orthopedic injuries.

The most crucial point in preventing injuries is not to overdo it. Even after you've been on the program for a while, never make a sudden large increase in the amount of exercise you perform. Always build your way up gradually.

In addition to gradual progression and warming up before each workout, wearing the right shoes is very important in preventing injury. Recent technological advances have resulted in shoes that not only are designed specifically for particular weight-bearing exercises but are also engineered to suit different types of feet. For example, some of you may have feet that "overpronate," or roll inward too much, on striking the ground. There are shoes made to negate this excessive foot motion. In contrast, others don't pronate enough. Because a certain degree of pronation is needed for adequate shock absorption, you would be better off with shoes that have good shock-absorbing properties.

A quality sporting goods or shoe store where the sales staff are well versed about athletic footgear is a good source for information about the correct shoe for your particular needs. There are several consumer fitness magazines containing annual shoe reviews which can also guide you to the appropriate shoe for the exercises you choose.

On a similar note, don't do weight-bearing exercises—particularly high-impact ones like jogging and jumping rope—day after day on hard, nonresistant surfaces. To ease the impact and stress on your musculoskeletal system, do these kinds of activities on grass or some other cushioned surface.

In the event that you do sustain an exercise-related orthopedic injury, keep in mind that the treatment you receive in the first 24 to 36 hours is key. During this period, you want not only to relieve pain but to limit swelling and inflammation that may interfere with the healing process. This is best accomplished by immediately starting a four-part first-aid program for exercise-related injuries known as RICE and continuing it for up to 36 hours.

1. R is for rest or reduce exercises that involve use of the injured body part. Continued exercise may ag-

gravate the injury. With serious injuries, days to weeks of rest or reduced training may be needed. To maintain health and fitness during this time, work around your injury by performing activities that don't require you to use the injured part of your body, just as Jimmy did while recovering from his wrist surgery. When pain-free activity is possible, make a gradual return to your usual routine.

2. I is for ice, which is applied to reduce swelling, bleeding, inflammation, and pain. Cold causes blood vessels at the site of the injury to contract and narrow, limiting bleeding and escape of fluid into the surrounding tissues. Crushed or chipped ice in plastic bags is one of the easiest ways to apply cold. The plastic bag should not be applied directly to the skin, as this could cause frostbite. Wrap the plastic bag in a towel or a sock before applying it to the injured part of the body. Ice should be applied for about 20 minutes each hour for the first three hours after the injury occurs. After that, two 20-minute applications each day will be adequate. Don't apply heat during the first 24 to 36 hours, as this may worsen swelling and inflammation.

3. C is for compression, which also helps limit swelling. If uncontrolled, swelling retards the healing process. For compression, wrap an elastic bandage firmly—but not so tightly that you shut off the blood supply—around the injured part. The bandage is too tight if you experience numbness, cramping, or pain. If any of these occur, unwrap the area immediately. Compression and ice can be applied at the same time by wrapping an ice-filled plastic bag within an elastic bandage around the injured area.

4. E is for elevation. Raise the injured body part above the level of the heart, allowing gravity to help drain excess fluid, which will reduce swelling. Place the elevated body part on a comfortable padded surface, such as a pillow.

Depending on the severity of your injury, you may also benefit from taking an over-the-counter anti-inflammatory medication. When doing so, be sure to read the directions carefully. Naturally, if you feel the injury is at all serious, see a doctor immediately.

6. Be cautious about exercising in adverse weather conditions—and know what precautions to take.

When you exercise, heat is one of the by-products of your working muscles. The more you exert yourself, of course, the more heat your body produces. Normally, sweating serves to remove excess heat from the body during exercise, preventing your temperature from rising too high. Hyperthermia, an overheating of the body while exercising, is something to be avoided. It not only impairs your ability to exercise but predisposes you to heat stroke, a potentially fatal condition.

The major symptoms of hyperthermia are headache, light-headedness, dizziness, confusion, disorientation, clumsiness, nausea, muscle cramps, hallucinations, and either excessive sweating or cessation of sweating altogether. You can avoid hyperthermia by taking these preventive measures:

• *Acclimatize your body to hot and humid weather conditions.* This can be done by gradually increasing the amount and intensity of your exercise in these conditions over a period of 10 to 14 days.

• *If you plan to exercise outdoors, take weather conditions into account.* Be sensible when heat and humidity are high. Don't engage in strenuous or prolonged exercise.

• *Be sure to drink fluids before and during exercise.* Even if you're not thirsty, you should drink about 8 ounces of cold water about 15 minutes before your workout begins. Cold water is absorbed more quickly than tepid water. If you exercise for longer than 30 minutes, take another 8-ounce drink at 15- to 20-minute intervals during exercise.

• *When exercising in warm weather, wear clothing that promotes heat loss.* Dress in loose-fitting, comfortable clothes made of porous material. People who are overweight sometimes work out in heavy clothing on purpose. They mistakenly think this will induce greater weight loss. What it does is create more sweating and fluid loss. The lost fluid must be replaced or dehydration will occur. Any weight loss at all will be very short-lived. In addition, wearing heavy clothing while working out increases the risk of hyperthermia. This is, in truth, the last thing you should do during warm- or hot-weather workouts.

• *When exercising in extreme heat, sponge off the exposed parts of your body—especially your active muscles—with cold water at 15- to 20-minute inter-*

vals. This will bring you instant relief and help lower your body temperature.

When dressing for a cold-weather workout, aim for adequate insulation while avoiding sweat buildup in your garments. This may sound like a contradictory proposition, but there is a solution. Wear multiple layers of clothing. Layered clothing has two main advantages. You can shed some of your clothes if you become too hot, and the layers will trap air in between, insulating your body from the cold. Unlike water, air is not a particularly good conductor of heat. Your innermost layer should serve to soak up excess sweat and carry it away from your skin. Recommended fabrics include polypropylene and cotton. Your middle layer of clothing should insulate; wool and goose-down garments will do this for you. On rainy, snowy, or very windy days, water-resistant materials such as Gore-Tex and nylon are the best choices for your outer clothing layer. Should you find that you get too warm in the middle of your workout, you may only need to unzip or unbutton this outer layer to get the desired cooling effect.

Since a lot of your body's heat can be lost through an uncovered head, wear a woolen cap or hooded sweatshirt when exercising outdoors. Gloves are also essential items when it comes to dressing for the outdoor workout.

Don't exercise outdoors if it's too cold, icy, or slippery. Obviously, falling on ice could cause severe injuries.

7. If at all possible, don't exercise in a heavily polluted environment.

Hot and cold weather aren't the only environmental hazards to consider. The quality of the air you breathe also has a measurable impact on your ability to work out safely. The U.S. Environmental Protection Agency singles out these most common pollutants: sulfur dioxide, carbon monoxide, nitrogen dioxide, ozone, hydrocarbons, lead, and total suspended particulates.

The two pollutants that probably pose the greatest threat to people who work out are carbon monoxide and ozone. Carbon monoxide, mostly contained in vehicle exhaust and cigarette smoke, interferes with the blood's ability to carry oxygen. Ozone, which is the result of a chemical reaction between automobile emissions and sunlight, irritates the lungs and may cause breathing problems.

To avoid excessive carbon monoxide exposure, don't work out along heavily traveled roadways during rush hour. Even if you are jogging, walking, or cycling on roads with light traffic, try to stay at least 20 yards away from passing vehicles, if possible. Naturally, you wouldn't want to work out in a smoke-filled room.

In order to avoid ozone, you should exercise at dawn or after the sun has set during the late spring and summer seasons, which is when sunlight is strongest. Ozone starts building up around 90 minutes after dawn and stops being generated at sunset, the peak concentration being at midday.

8. Don't work out when you have the flu or any other illness that is associated with a fever.

If you've got nothing more serious than a slight cold, you can go ahead with your workout provided your temperature is normal, your symptoms are above the neck (i.e., sneezing, runny nose, scratchy throat), and, of course, you feel like it. But when your ailment is more serious, and especially if it's accompanied by a fever, you'd better sit out aerobic exercise and all other forms of strenuous exercise until you're better. Infectious fever and strenuous exercise are a bad combination. They can trigger hyperthermia, worsen the infection, and even place you at risk for a potentially lethal inflammatory condition of the heart muscle called viral myocarditis.

Before resuming exercise after a flu-like illness, wait until your body temperature has been normal for at least 48 hours. Then return to your usual level of physical activity gradually, over the course of a week or two. *Never* attempt to "sweat out" a fever.

9. Follow proper exercise protocol when performing muscle-strengthening exercises.

Be sure to maintain good posture and use the correct technique when performing muscle-strengthening exercises. If you are unable to do this, the weight or resistance you are using might be too great for your current strength level and should be reduced.

Avoid holding your breath during muscle-strengthening exercises, for this places unnecessary stress on your cardiovascular system. If you feel inclined to do so, it could be another indicator that the weight or resistance you're using is too challenging for your current strength level and is forcing you to strain excessively. As a general rule, you should try to exhale during the effort part of each movement, while lifting, pushing, or pulling.

10. Don't work out infrequently.

Exercising infrequently is a mistake. By doing so, you don't give your body a chance to adapt to your workouts. When you do finally exercise again, you expose yourself to the risk of injury without the possibility of getting the benefits from your previous session. Don't be a weekend, once-a-month, or holiday fitness buff. Strive to work out at least 3 times per week.

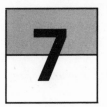

7

16 Weeks to a Lifetime of Fitness

IT IS TIME to begin the Jimmy Connors Workout. I am convinced beyond a shadow of a doubt that you will love my program like no other program you may have tried or read about before. I promise that the results you experience will change the way you view everything else in your life. But it is important to me that you enjoy the process of the change you are about to make rather than just wait anxiously for the end of the 16 weeks. If all you cared about was the results, the enjoyment of the program itself would be lost in your anticipation. Life is too damn short to waste even 4 months. Besides, the 16-week period is only the beginning. At the end of that time you should be comfortable doing all the exercises and be able to continue forever with the program for maintenance purposes.

HOW TO USE THE PROGRAM

- *Decide which of my two programs is best for you.*

Program A is for those who either have never exercised regularly (20 minutes a day on at least 3 days of the week) or have not been doing so for 4 months or more.

Program B was created for those who already work out for 20 minutes or longer on at least 3 days a week, have been following this routine for at least 4 months, and like a more strenuous workout. This one is for physically active people who want to take their degree of fitness to a higher level.

If you do work out on a regular basis but are not interested in a strenuous program, you have another alternative. You can do Program A, beginning in Week 4. Once you've finished Week 16, continue for an additional 4 weeks with the Program A 4-Week Optional Extension. This will provide those of you who are not strangers to exercise with the maximum amount of exercise you need without its being too strenuous.

Although you have been given two different programs from which to choose, they are both adapted from my personal workout. I do precisely these exercises regularly but at a higher level of intensity because I am a professional athlete. When I decide to give up pro tennis, I will do these exercises at a lower intensity for the rest of my life, just as I'm suggesting you do.

- *Once you've decided on a program, read each day's suggestions carefully.*

In each workout program I have provided detailed instructions on how much aerobic exercise and strength training should be performed on each day. I have not included stretching guidelines because they are the same throughout each program. You should perform two to three gentle repetitions of the stretching exercises shown in Figures 7-1 to 7-5 after each aerobic workout.

- *Exercise your options.*

The exercises listed on the programs are my choices, what I do during my workouts. If you like these choices, great. But if you would rather perform other exercises or just one of them, that's OK too. There are many exercises you can do instead of mine which will give you the same results. For each of my choices, I have listed on pages 211–12 two sets of options—one set for low-intensity exercises, the other for moderate- to high-intensity exercises. Think of it as the Jimmy Connors Workout tailor-made for you.

HOW TO CALCULATE YOUR POINTS ON THE CONNORS COUNT

Working with the Connors Count is very easy. For each activity you do, keep track of the number of minutes you did it along with your rating of perceived exertion

(RPE) on the Borg Scale. Then go to the Connors Count Index on pages 192–195 where you'll find the activity and its corresponding RPE level; you will then be referred to one of 14 (A–N) charts on pages 196–209, where the Connors Count points will be calculated for you according to the amount of time you spent doing each activity.

Let's say I played racquetball at an RPE of 12 for 45 minutes. I look up racquetball on the Connors Count Index and see that because I played at an RPE of 12, I'm referred to Chart J. On Chart J, I find that the number of points I've earned for 45 minutes of play is 24.3.

At the end of each day, add up the number of points you've earned for each bout of exercise and round the total off to the nearest whole number. At the end of the week, take your total points and refer to page 213, where you can check out the effectiveness of the entire week's worth of activity.

Example 1

Walking 10 minutes at an RPE below 12 = 1.8 points.

If this accounted for all the exercise you did on a given day, you'd round off the 1.8 to 2 and your Connors Count for the day would be 2.

Example 2

Walking 3 minutes at an RPE below 12 = 0.5 point (your warm-up).

Walking 17 minutes at an RPE of 13 = 6.1 points.

Stationary cycle (dual-action) 17 minutes at an RPE of 12 = 8.2 points.

Stationary cycle (dual-action) 3 minutes at an RPE below 12 = 0.6 point (your cool-down).

If this was your day's physical activity, the sum of your earned points would be 15.4. You'd then round off that figure to 15, which would be your total of Connors Count points for the day.

• *Note:*

If you choose an activity which is not listed on the index, you can still get a pretty good idea of how many points you've earned by finding on the index another activity you think is very similar and then using the charts in the same way. Remember, when noting the time of your exercise sessions, that if you're doing an activity that calls for a lot of starts and stops, as long as the stops don't last for longer than a minute, you can take credit for the entire duration. But if you're playing tennis, let's say, and every time you and your partner go to pick up balls, you stand and chat at the net for a few minutes, you can only count the time you actually spent playing.

I have no way of knowing how many points you already have earned on the Connors Count as a result of the activities you do in your daily life. Because of this, I designed my programs assuming you did only the scheduled exercises in the program of your choice. I'm sure that's not the case for most of you.

I recommend that you keep track of all bouts of exercise you do throughout the day, especially those that last longer than 2 minutes. By all means, credit yourself with points for these activities and cut back accordingly on my exercise recommendations.

For example, if during the day you put in 5 minutes of walking upstairs at an RPE of 12 (which would earn you 2.1 points) and another 10 minutes of walking to and from lunch at an RPE of less than 12 (1.8 points), you have already earned 4 points on the Connors Count. If your scheduled workout for that day normally included 30 minutes of brisk walking at an RPE of 13 (11 points), you could cut back to 20 minutes (7.2 points) and still earn the same amount of points for that day. If you climbed the stairs and walked to and from lunch on 3 days during the week, you could cut out an entire 30-minute workout! Why do more than you need to?

It is up to you to decide whether you want to earn 35 points, 100 points, or somewhere in the middle each week. Keep in mind that the closer you get to 100, the more benefit you'll receive, but if you decide that 35 points is enough for you, that's fine. When using Program A, you don't have to go further than Week 7 to get those 35 points. After that you would just keep doing Week 7 to maintain the benefits and possibly substitute different exercises for variation. If you change your mind later on and want the challenge of earning more points, you can pick up at Week 8 of Program A anytime as long as you didn't stop exercising completely.

Although 100 points is the highest number you need to strive for, many experts consider 75 points to be plenty. This is why Program A stops at 75 points. If you want to go for the entire 100 points without taking on the strenuous level of Program B, the Program A 4-Week Optional Extension will give you the 25 extra points needed without working you too hard.

I consider the Jimmy Connors Program A to be the best for most men and women over the age of 35. It involves low-impact activities that can be done easily with a very low risk of injury. However, those of you who are used to or would like to become used to a tougher workout will find enough challenge in Program B. Be aware that although this is an excellent workout, it does come with a slightly higher risk of injury. Remember to listen to your body and either slow down or switch to another exercise if you should feel any pain in your muscles and/or joints.

Finally, don't try to rush the program. Neil and I chose 16 weeks because we felt that it was long enough to acclimate you safely to a new routine and yet short enough to give you dramatic results relatively fast. If, on the other hand, you want to repeat a week or two, that's not a problem. Take as long as you want to reach your goal. Just don't give up and, I guarantee, you won't be sorry.

Program A

	MONDAY	**TUESDAY**	**WEDNESDAY**
W **E** **E** **K** **1**	AEROBICS • Walk 5 min. at RPE <12 (see Options 1).		AEROBICS • Walk 7 min. at RPE <12 (see Options 1).
	CONNORS COUNT = 1		CONNORS COUNT = 1

COMMENTS

• Congratulations! Making up your mind to get started is often the hardest part about changing any lifestyle behavior.
• Your first few workouts should feel so easy that you think I'm wasting your time.
• During the first 5 weeks of your aerobics program, the emphasis is on

THURSDAY	FRIDAY	SATURDAY	SUNDAY

AEROBICS
• Walk 10 min.
at RPE <12 (see
Options 1).

CONNORS
COUNT
= 2

gradually increasing the length of time you can exercise. Don't worry
about whether the exercise is intense enough for you or not—just
choose an intensity that feels comfortable to you and does not cause
you to rate your exertion above a 12 on the Borg Scale.
• Remember to stretch after each workout.

**WEEK 1
CONNORS
COUNT
= 4**

	MONDAY	**TUESDAY**	**WEDNESDAY**
W **E** **E** **K** **2**	AEROBICS • Walk 12 min. at RPE <12 (see Options 1). STRENGTHENING • 1 set of 8 reps of 10 exercises. Select weight/resistance so that RPE <12.		AEROBICS • Walk 15 min. at RPE <12 (see Options 1).
	CONNORS COUNT = 3		CONNORS COUNT = 3

COMMENTS

• You may feel a little sore after your first few muscle-strengthening sessions. Provided it is not too severe, this "delayed onset muscle soreness" is quite normal and should disappear completely within a week or two after starting any new exercise.

• Consider using my home muscle-strengthening program (see the photo insert).

• If you rest for 60 seconds or less between each set of resistance exer-

AEROBICS
- Walk 17 min. at RPE <12 (see Options 1).

STRENGTHENING
- 1 set of 10 reps of 10 exercises. Use same weight/resistance; keep RPE <12.

CONNORS
COUNT
= 4

cises you are performing what is known as "circuit training" and can count it toward the Connors Count. I suggest that you credit yourself with 0.5 minute of circuit training for each set of muscle-strengthening exercises.
- If the weight/resistance you choose elicits an RPE above 12, it is too heavy for you at this stage of your program.

**WEEK 2
CONNORS
COUNT
= 10**

	MONDAY	TUESDAY	WEDNESDAY
W E E K 3	**AEROBICS** • Walk 20 min. at RPE <12 (see Options 1). **STRENGTHENING** • 1 set of 12 reps of 10 exercises. Use same weight/resistance; keep RPE <12.		**AEROBICS** • Walk 20 min. at RPE <12 (see Options 1). • Stationary cycle (dual-action) 5 min. at RPE <12 (see Options 1).
	CONNORS COUNT = 5		CONNORS COUNT = 5

COMMENTS

• Now that you've worked your way up to 20 minutes of walking it's time to add in a second aerobic activity.

• When starting any new aerobic activity, begin slowly and increase your exercise time gradually.

• Remember, you do have choices. So if stationary cycling is not to your

AEROBICS
- Walk 20 min. at RPE <12 (see Options 1).
- Stationary cycle (dual-action) 7 min. at RPE <12 (see Options 1).

STRENGTHENING
- 1 set of 12 reps of 10 exercises. Use same weight/resistance; keep RPE <12.

CONNORS
COUNT
= 6

liking, select one of the other options. Or even use walking as your only aerobic activity should you wish to.
- Don't forget to perform 2 to 3 gentle repetitions of the stretching exercises shown in the photo insert after each workout.

**WEEK 3
CONNORS
COUNT
= 16**

	MONDAY	TUESDAY	WEDNESDAY
W E E K 4	**AEROBICS** • Walk 20 min. at RPE <12 (see Options 1). • Stationary cycle (dual-action) 10 min. at RPE <12 (see Options 1). **STRENGTHENING** • 1 set of 8 reps of 9 exercises + 14 sit-ups. Increase weight/resistance; keep RPE <12.		**AEROBICS** • Walk 20 min. at RPE <12 (see Options 1). • Stationary cycle (dual-action) 12 min. at RPE <12 (see Options 1).
	CONNORS COUNT = 7		CONNORS COUNT = 6

COMMENTS

• Keep it up. You're progressing well. Although you are only in your 4th week of my program, you are already doing over 30 minutes of aerobic exercise during each workout.

THURSDAY	FRIDAY	SATURDAY	SUNDAY
	AEROBICS		

AEROBICS
• Walk 20 min. at RPE <12 (see Options 1).
• Stationary cycle (dual-action) 15 min. at RPE <12 (see Options 1).

STRENGTHENING
• 1 set of 8 reps of 9 exercises + 14 sit-ups. Use same weight/resistance; keep RPE <12.

CONNORS
COUNT
= 8

• It's time to increase the weight/resistance you are using during strength training. When doing so, drop your number of repetitions back down to 8 and keep your RPE below 12.

**WEEK 4
CONNORS
COUNT
= 21**

	MONDAY	TUESDAY	WEDNESDAY
W E E K 5	**AEROBICS** • Walk 20 min. at RPE <12 (see Options 1). • Stationary cycle (dual-action) 17 min. at RPE <12 (see Options 1). **STRENGTHENING** • 1 set of 10 reps of 9 exercises + 16 sit-ups. Use same weight/resistance; keep RPE <12.		**AEROBICS** • Walk 20 min. at RPE <12 (see Options 1). • Stationary cycle (dual-action) 20 min. at RPE <12 (see Options 1).
	CONNORS COUNT = 8		**CONNORS COUNT = 8**

COMMENTS

• Well done! You've worked your way up to 40 minutes of aerobic exercise. You are now ready to move on to moderately intense exercise, which is what I recommend to improve both the functional-fitness and the health-promotion components of your health-related fitness level.

THURSDAY	FRIDAY	SATURDAY	SUNDAY
	AEROBICS • Walk 20 min. at RPE <12 (see Options 1). • Stationary cycle (dual-action) 20 min. at RPE <12 (see Options 1). STRENGTHENING • 1 set of 10 reps of 9 exercises + 16 sit-ups. Use same weight/resistance; keep RPE <12.		
	CONNORS COUNT = 9		
			WEEK 5 CONNORS COUNT = 25

	MONDAY	TUESDAY	WEDNESDAY

W E E K 6

MONDAY	TUESDAY	WEDNESDAY
AEROBICS • Walk 17 min. at RPE <12; 3 min. at RPE = 12–13 (see Options 1). • Stationary cycle (dual-action) 20 min. at RPE <12 (see Options 1). STRENGTHENING • 1 set of 12 reps of 9 exercises + 18 sit-ups. Use same weight/resistance; keep RPE <12.		AEROBICS • Walk 17 min. at RPE <12; 3 min. at RPE = 12–13 (see Options 1). • Stationary cycle (dual-action) 3 min. at RPE = 12–13; 17 min. at RPE <12 (see Options 1).
CONNORS COUNT = 9		CONNORS COUNT = 9

COMMENTS

• Your body—in particular, its musculoskeletal and cardiorespiratory systems—is now accustomed to prolonged, low-intensity aerobic exercise. Now it's time to gradually introduce moderate-intensity exercise into your program.

• Should you wish to stay with low-intensity aerobic exercise, that's OK.

AEROBICS
• Walk 15 min.
at RPE <12; 5
min at RPE =
12–13 (see Options 1).
• Stationary
cycle (dual-action) 3 min. at
RPE = 12–13; 17
min. at RPE <12
(see Options 1).

STRENGTHENING
• 1 set of 12
reps of 9 exercises + 18 sit-ups. Use same
weight/resistance; keep RPE
<12.

CONNORS
COUNT
= 10

To earn my minimum recommended number of points on the Connors Count (35), you will need to increase your exercise time and/or work out more frequently. Although this will benefit your health and promote weight loss, it probably won't have a major impact on your functional fitness level.

**WEEK 6
CONNORS
COUNT
= 28**

	MONDAY	TUESDAY	WEDNESDAY
W E E K 7	**AEROBICS** • Walk 15 min. at RPE <12; 5 min. at RPE = 12–13 (see Options 1). • Stationary cycle (dual-action) 5 min. at RPE = 12–13; 15 min at RPE <12 (see Options 1). **STRENGTHENING** • 1 set of 12 reps of 9 exercises + 20 sit-ups. Use same weight/resistance; keep RPE <12. • 1 set of 8 reps of 10 exercises. Select weight/resistance so that RPE = 12–15. **CONNORS COUNT = 13**		**AEROBICS** • Walk 15 min. at RPE <12; 5 min at RPE = 12–13 (see Options 1). • Stationary cycle (dual-action) 5 min. at RPE = 12–13; 15 min. at RPE <12 (see Options 1). **CONNORS COUNT = 10**

COMMENTS

• Hey, you're already above 35 points on the Connors Count. This is the minimum amount of weekly aerobic exercise recommended by the American Heart Association.

• You've also now added a second set of muscle-strengthening exercises, which you are doing with a weight/resistance that feels like a 12–15 on the Borg Scale to you (credit yourself with an additional 0.5 minute of circuit training per exercise when tallying your Connors Count).

AEROBICS
- Walk 15 min. at RPE <12; 5 min. at RPE = 12–13 (see Options 1).
- Stationary cycle (dual-action) 5 min. at RPE = 12–13; 15 min. at RPE <12 (see Options 1).

STRENGTHENING
- 1 set of 12 reps of 9 exercises + 20 sit-ups. Use same weight/resistance; keep RPE <12.
- 1 set of 8 reps of 10 exercises. Select weight/resistance so that RPE = 12–15.

CONNORS
COUNT
= 13

- Use the first set of each exercise as a warm-up set to reduce your risk of injury.
- You are now getting more than the minimum amount of strength training recommended by the American College of Sports Medicine.

**WEEK 7
CONNORS
COUNT
= 36**

	MONDAY	**TUESDAY**	**WEDNESDAY**
W E E K 8	AEROBICS • Walk 13 min. at RPE <12; 7 min. at RPE = 12–13 (see Options 1). • Stationary cycle (dual-action) 5 min. at RPE = 12–13; 15 min. at RPE <12 (see Options 1). STRENGTHENING • 1 set of 12 reps of 9 exercises + 20 sit-ups. Use same weight/re-sistance; keep RPE <12. • 1 set of 10 reps of 9 exercises + 10 sit-ups. Use same weight/re-sistance; keep RPE = 12–15. CONNORS COUNT = 13		AEROBICS • Walk 13 min. at RPE <12; 7 min. at RPE = 12–13 (see Options 1). • Stationary cycle (dual-action) 7 min. at RPE = 12–13; 13 min. at RPE <12 (see Options 1). CONNORS COUNT = 11

COMMENTS

• If you are comfortable getting the minimum amount of exercise to promote your health-related fitness level, simply continue with Week 7's workouts. Be proud of yourself—fewer than 10 percent of adult Americans exercise this amount on a regular basis.

AEROBICS
- Walk 10 min. at RPE <12; 10 min. at RPE = 12–13 (see Options 1).
- Stationary cycle (dual-action) 7 min. at RPE = 12–13; 13 min. at RPE <12 (see Options 1).

STRENGTHENING
- 1 set of 12 reps of 9 exercises + 20 sit-ups. Use same weight/resistance; keep RPE <12.
- 1 set of 10 reps of 9 exercises + 10 sit-ups. Use same weight/resistance; keep RPE = 12–15.

CONNORS COUNT = 14

- However, if you're not satisfied with the bare minimum, it's time to start working toward 50 points on the Connors Count.

WEEK 8 CONNORS COUNT = 38

	MONDAY	TUESDAY	WEDNESDAY
W E E K 9	**AEROBICS** • Walk 10 min. at RPE <12; 10 min. at RPE = 12–13 (see Options 1). • Stationary cycle (dual-action) 10 min. at RPE = 12–13; 10 min. at RPE <12 (see Options 1). **STRENGTHENING** • 1 set of 12 reps of 9 exercises + 20 sit-ups. Use same weight/resistance; keep RPE <12. • 1 set of 12 reps of 9 exercises + 12 sit-ups. Use same weight/resistance; keep RPE = 12–15. **CONNORS COUNT = 15**		**AEROBICS** • Walk 7 min. at RPE <12; 13 min. at RPE = 12–13 (see Options 1). • Stationary cycle (dual-action) 10 min. at RPE = 12–13; 10 min. at RPE <12 (see Options 1). **CONNORS COUNT = 13**

COMMENTS

• Be patient, it won't be long before you are doing all of your aerobic workouts at a moderate intensity.

THURSDAY	FRIDAY	SATURDAY	SUNDAY

AEROBICS
- Walk 7 min. at RPE <12; 13 min. at RPE = 12–13 (see Options 1).
- Stationary cycle (dual-action) 13 min. at RPE = 12–13; 7 min. at RPE <12 (see Options 1).

STRENGTHENING
- 1 set of 12 reps of 9 exercises + 20 sit-ups. Use same weight/resistance; keep RPE <12.
- 1 set of 12 reps of 9 exercises + 12 sit-ups. Use same weight/resistance; keep RPE = 12–15.

CONNORS COUNT = 16

WEEK 9 CONNORS COUNT = 44

	MONDAY	**TUESDAY**	**WEDNESDAY**
W E E K 10	**AEROBICS** • Walk 5 min. at RPE <12; 15 min. at RPE = 12–13 (see Options 1). • Stationary cycle (dual-action) 13 min. at RPE = 12–13; 7 min. at RPE <12 (see Options 1). **STRENGTHENING** • 1 set of 12 reps of 9 exercises + 20 sit-ups. Use same weight/resistance; keep RPE <12. • 1 set of 8 reps of 9 exercises + 14 sit-ups. Increase weight/resistance; keep RPE = 12–15. **CONNORS COUNT = 16**		**AEROBICS** • Walk 5 min. at RPE <12; 15 min. at RPE = 12–13 (see Options 1). • Stationary cycle (dual-action) 15 min. at RPE = 12–13; 5 min. at RPE <12 (see Options 1). **CONNORS COUNT = 15**

COMMENTS

• It's time to up the weight/resistance for your second set of muscle-strengthening exercises. When doing so, reduce the number of repetitions to 8 and keep your RPE at 12–15. There is no need to increase the weight/resistance for your first set of each exercise; remember, it's intended as a warm-up.

THURSDAY	FRIDAY	SATURDAY	SUNDAY

AEROBICS
- Walk 3 min. at RPE < 12; 17 min. at RPE = 12–13 (see Options 1).
- Stationary cycle (dual-action) 15 min. at RPE = 12–13; 5 min. at RPE < 12 (see Options 1).

STRENGTHENING
- 1 set of 12 reps of 9 exercises + 20 sit-ups. Use same weight/resistance; keep RPE < 12.
- 1 set of 8 reps of 9 exercises + 14 sit-ups. Use same weight/resistance; keep RPE = 12–15.

CONNORS COUNT = 17

WEEK 10 CONNORS COUNT = 48

	MONDAY	TUESDAY	WEDNESDAY

W E E K 11

MONDAY

AEROBICS
 • Walk 3 min. at RPE <12; 17 min. at RPE = 12–13 (see Options 1).
 • Stationary cycle (dual-action) 17 min. at RPE = 12–13; 3 min. at RPE <12 (see Options 1).

STRENGTHENING
 • 1 set of 12 reps of 9 exercises + 20 sit-ups. Use same weight/resistance; keep RPE <12.
 • 1 set of 10 reps of 9 exercises + 16 sit-ups. Use same weight/resistance; keep RPE = 12–15.

CONNORS COUNT = 18

WEDNESDAY

AEROBICS
 • Walk 3 min. at RPE <12; 17 min. at RPE = 12–13 (see Options 1).
 • Stationary cycle (dual-action) 17 min. at RPE = 12–13; 3 min. at RPE <12 (see Options 1).

CONNORS COUNT = 15

COMMENTS

 • This is an important week in the Jimmy Connors Workout Program. You've not only exceeded 50 points on the Connors Count, but you are now getting most of these points from moderate-intensity exercise. The 3 minutes of aerobic exercise at an RPE below 12 at the beginning and end

THURSDAY	FRIDAY	SATURDAY	SUNDAY

AEROBICS
- Walk 3 min. at RPE <12; 17 min. at RPE = 12–13 (see Options 1).
- Stationary cycle (dual-action) 17 min. at RPE = 12–13; 3 min. at RPE <12 (see Options 1).

STRENGTHENING
- 1 set of 12 reps of 9 exercises + 20 sit-ups. Use same weight/resistance; keep RPE <12.
- 1 set of 10 reps of 9 exercises + 16 sit-ups. Use same weight/resistance; keep RPE = 12–15.

CONNORS COUNT = 18

of each aerobic workout are intended as a warm-up and cool-down; however, you still take credit for them when using the Connors Count.

WEEK 11 CONNORS COUNT = 51

	MONDAY	TUESDAY	WEDNESDAY

W E E K 12

MONDAY

AEROBICS
• Walk 3 min. at RPE <12; 17 min. at RPE = 12–13 (see Options 1).
• Stationary cycle (dual-action) 17 min. at RPE = 12–13; 3 min. at RPE <12 (see Options 1).

STRENGTHENING
• 1 set of 12 reps of 9 exercises + 20 sit-ups. Use same weight/resistance; keep RPE <12.
• 1 set of 12 reps of 9 exercises + 18 sit-ups. Use same weight/resistance; keep RPE = 12–15.

CONNORS COUNT = 18

WEDNESDAY

AEROBICS
• Walk 3 min. at RPE <12; 17 min. at RPE = 12–13 (see Options 1).
• Stationary cycle (dual-action) 17 min. at RPE = 12–13; 3 min. at RPE <12 (see Options 1).

CONNORS COUNT = 15

COMMENTS

• If you don't want to spend any more of your time on exercise, be happy with 50 points on the Connors Count and continue with Week 11's workouts.

• If you are prepared to invest a bit more time and effort in your health and fitness, then set your sights on 75 points. One way to get there is to

THURSDAY	FRIDAY	SATURDAY	SUNDAY
	AEROBICS • Walk 3 min. at RPE <12; 17 min. at RPE = 12–13 (see Options 1). • Stationary cycle (dual-action) 17 min. at RPE = 12–13; 3 min. at RPE <12 (see Options 1). **STRENGTHENING** • 1 set of 12 reps of 9 exercises + 20 sit-ups. Use same weight/resistance; keep RPE <12. • 1 set of 12 reps of 9 exercises + 18 sit-ups. Use same weight/resistance; keep RPE = 12–15. CONNORS COUNT = 18	**AEROBICS** • Walk 3 min. at RPE <12; 15 min. at RPE = 12–13; 3 min. at RPE <12 (see Options 1). CONNORS COUNT = 7	

exercise more frequently, which is why I'm recommending that you add an extra day to your program at this stage. If you choose a new activity for this extra day, you should introduce it more gradually into your program.

WEEK 12 CONNORS COUNT = 58

	MONDAY	TUESDAY	WEDNESDAY
W E E K 13	**AEROBICS** • Walk 3 min. at RPE <12; 17 min. at RPE = 12–13 (see Options 1). • Stationary cycle (dual-action) 17 min. at RPE = 12–13; 3 min. at RPE <12 (see Options 1). **STRENGTHENING** • 1 set of 12 reps of 9 exercises + 20 sit-ups. Use same weight/resistance; keep RPE <12. • 1 set of 8 reps of 9 exercises + 20 sit-ups. Increase weight/resistance; keep RPE = 12–15. **CONNORS COUNT = 18**		**AEROBICS** • Walk 3 min. at RPE <12; 17 min. at RPE = 12–13 (see Options 1). • Stationary cycle (dual-action) 17 min. at RPE = 12–13; 3 min. at RPE <12 (see Options 1). **CONNORS COUNT = 15**

COMMENTS

• You should be used to the routine by now. Provided 12 repetitions did not feel too hard for you to complete, you can increase the weight/resistance you have been using for your second set of muscle-strengthening exercises and reduce your repetitions to 8 again.

THURSDAY	FRIDAY	SATURDAY	SUNDAY

FRIDAY

AEROBICS
- Walk 3 min. at RPE <12; 17 min. at RPE = 12–13 (see Options 1).
- Stationary cycle (dual-action) 17 min. at RPE = 12–13; 3 min. at RPE <12 (see Options 1).

STRENGTHENING
- 1 set of 12 reps of 9 exercises + 20 sit-ups. Use same weight/resistance; keep RPE <12.
- 1 set of 8 reps of 9 exercises + 20 sit-ups. Use same weight/resistance; keep RPE = 12–15.

CONNORS COUNT = 18

SATURDAY

AEROBICS
- Walk 3 min. at RPE <12; 20 min. at RPE = 12–13; 3 min. at RPE <12 (see Options 1).

CONNORS COUNT = 8

WEEK 13 CONNORS COUNT = 59

	MONDAY	TUESDAY	WEDNESDAY
W E E K 14	**AEROBICS** • Walk 3 min. at RPE <12; 17 min. at RPE = 12–13 (see Options 1). • Stationary cycle (dual-action) 17 min. at RPE = 12–13; 3 min. at RPE <12 (see Options 1). **STRENGTHENING** • 1 set of 12 reps of 9 exercises + 20 sit-ups. Use same weight/resistance; keep RPE <12. • 1 set of 10 reps of 9 exercises + 20 sit-ups. Use same weight/resistance; keep RPE = 12–15. **CONNORS COUNT = 18**	**AEROBICS** • Walk 3 min. at RPE <12; 20 min. at RPE = 12–13; 3 min. at RPE <12 (see Options 1). **CONNORS COUNT = 8**	**AEROBICS** • Walk 3 min. at RPE <12; 17 min. at RPE = 12–13 (see Options 1). • Stationary cycle (dual-action) 17 min. at RPE = 12–13; 3 min. at RPE <12 (see Options 1). **CONNORS COUNT = 15**

COMMENTS

• I recommend adding a 5th day of exercise at this point. However, if you prefer to stay with 4 days per week, you can; rather than exercising more frequently, you can increase the duration of your aerobic workouts on the days you already train.

THURSDAY	FRIDAY	SATURDAY	SUNDAY

FRIDAY

AEROBICS
• Walk 3 min. at RPE <12; 17 min. at RPE = 12–13 (see Options 1).
• Stationary cycle (dual-action) 17 min. at RPE = 12–13; 3 min. at RPE <12 (see Options 1).

STRENGTHENING
• 1 set of 12 reps of 9 exercises + 20 sit-ups. Use same weight/resistance; keep RPE <12.
• 1 set of 10 reps of 9 exercises + 20 sit-ups. Use same weight/resistance; keep RPE = 12–15.

CONNORS COUNT = 18

SATURDAY

AEROBICS
• Walk 3 min. at RPE <12; 20 min. at RPE = 12–13; 3 min. at RPE <12 (see Options 1).

CONNORS COUNT = 8

WEEK 14 CONNORS COUNT = 67

	MONDAY	TUESDAY	WEDNESDAY
W E E K 15	**AEROBICS** • Walk 3 min. at RPE <12; 17 min. at RPE = 12–13 (see Options 1). • Stationary cycle (dual-action) 17 min. at RPE = 12–13; 3 min. at RPE <12 (see Options 1). **STRENGTHENING** • 1 set of 12 reps of 9 exercises + 20 sit-ups. Use same weight/resistance; keep RPE <12. • 1 set of 12 reps of 9 exercises + 20 sit-ups. Use same weight/resistance; keep RPE = 12–13.	**AEROBICS** • Walk 3 min. at RPE <12; 25 min. at RPE = 12–13; 3 min. at RPE <12 (see Options 1).	**AEROBICS** • Walk 3 min. at RPE <12; 17 min. at RPE = 12–13 (see Options 1). • Stationary cycle (dual-action) 17 min. at RPE = 12–13; 3 min. at RPE <12 (see Options 1).
	CONNORS COUNT = 18	CONNORS COUNT = 10	CONNORS COUNT = 15

COMMENTS

• Your persistence has paid off. Next week you will reach 75 on the Connors Count.

THURSDAY	FRIDAY	SATURDAY	SUNDAY
	AEROBICS • Walk 3 min. at RPE <12; 17 min. at RPE = 12–13 (see Options 1). • Stationary cycle (dual-action) 17 min. at RPE = 12–13; 3 min. at RPE <12 (see Options 1). STRENGTHENING • 1 set of 12 reps of 9 exercises + 20 sit-ups. Use same weight/resistance; keep RPE <12. • 1 set of 12 reps of 9 exercises + 20 sit-ups. Use same weight/resistance; keep RPE = 12–13. CONNORS COUNT = 18	AEROBICS • Walk 3 min. at RPE <12; 25 min. at RPE = 12–13; 3 min. at RPE <12 (see Options 1). CONNORS COUNT = 10	

WEEK 15 CONNORS COUNT = 71

	MONDAY	TUESDAY	WEDNESDAY
WEEK 16 AND ONWARD	**AEROBICS** • Walk 3 min. at RPE <12; 17 min. at RPE = 12–13 (see Options 1). • Stationary cycle (dual-action) 17 min. at RPE = 12–13; 3 min. at RPE <12 (see Options 1). **STRENGTHENING** • 1 set of 12 reps of 9 exercises + 20 sit-ups. Use same weight/resistance; keep RPE <12. • 1 set of 12 reps of 9 exercises + 20 sit-ups. Use same weight/resistance; keep RPE = 12–15.	**AEROBICS** • Walk 3 min. at RPE <12; 30 min. at RPE = 12–13; 3 min. at RPE <12 (see Options 1).	**AEROBICS** • Walk 3 min. at RPE <12; 17 min. at RPE = 12–13 (see Options 1). • Stationary cycle (dual-action) 17 min. at RPE = 12–13; 3 min. at RPE <12 (see Options 1).
	CONNORS COUNT = 18	**CONNORS COUNT = 12**	**CONNORS COUNT = 15**

COMMENTS

• Just as I told you—you did it! Congratulations—you didn't allow yourself to be counted out. Many health and fitness experts consider this to be an ideal amount of exercise. By now you've dramatically improved your level of health-related fitness. You now have three options: (1) Stick with Week 16's program and you will not only maintain these benefits but continue to derive additional ones. (2) Use the 4-Week Optional Extension

THURSDAY	FRIDAY	SATURDAY	SUNDAY
	AEROBICS • Walk 3 min. at RPE <12; 17 min. at RPE = 12–13 (see Options 1). • Stationary cycle (dual-action) 17 min. at RPE = 12–13; 3 min. at RPE <12 (see Options 1). STRENGTHENING • 1 set of 12 reps of 9 exercises + 20 sit-ups. Use same weight/resistance; keep RPE <12. • 1 set of 12 reps of 9 exercises + 20 sit-ups. Use same weight/resistance; keep RPE = 12–15. CONNORS COUNT = 18	AEROBICS • Walk 3 min. at RPE <12; 30 min. at RPE = 12–13; 3 min. at RPE <12 (see Options 1). CONNORS COUNT = 12	

to reach 100 points per week. (3) If you prefer more strenuous workouts move on to Program B. When doing so, continue with your same strengthening workouts and start with Week 3's aerobic workouts (don't be concerned about earning fewer than 75 points in the beginning).

**WEEK 16
CONNORS
COUNT
= 75**

Jimmy Connors Workout Program A
4-Week Optional Extension

	MONDAY	TUESDAY	WEDNESDAY
W			
E			
E			
K			
17			

MONDAY	TUESDAY	WEDNESDAY
AEROBICS • Walk 3 min. at RPE <12; 17 min. at RPE = 12–13 (see Options 1). • Stationary cycle (dual-action) 20 min. at RPE = 12–13; 3 min. at RPE <12 (see Options 1). STRENGTHENING • 1 set of 12 reps of 9 exercises + 20 sit-ups. Use same weight/resistance; keep RPE <12. • 1 set of 12 reps of 9 exercises + 20 sit-ups. Use same weight/resistance; keep RPE = 12–15.	AEROBICS • Walk 3 min. at RPE <12; 30 min. at RPE = 12–13; 3 min. at RPE <12 (see Options 1).	AEROBICS • Walk 3 min. at RPE <12; 17 min. at RPE = 12–13 (see Options 1). • Stationary cycle (dual-action) 20 min. at RPE = 12–13; 3 min. at RPE <12 (see Options 1).
CONNORS COUNT = 19	CONNORS COUNT = 12	CONNORS COUNT = 17

COMMENTS

• Over the course of the next 4 weeks I am going to help you modify your program slightly so that you reach 100 points on the Connors Count. It won't take that much more effort.

THURSDAY	FRIDAY	SATURDAY	SUNDAY
	AEROBICS • Walk 3 min. at RPE <12; 17 min. at RPE = 12–13 (see Options 1). • Stationary cycle (dual-action) 20 min. at RPE = 12–13; 3 min. at RPE <12 (see Options 1). **STRENGTHENING** • 1 set of 12 reps of 9 exercises + 20 sit-ups. Use same weight/resistance; keep RPE <12. • 1 set of 12 reps of 9 exercises + 20 sit-ups. Use same weight/resistance; keep RPE = 12–15. CONNORS COUNT = 19	**AEROBICS** • Walk 3 min. at RPE <12; 30 min. at RPE = 12–13; 3 min. at RPE <12 (see Options 1). CONNORS COUNT = 12	

WEEK 17 CONNORS COUNT = 79

	MONDAY	TUESDAY	WEDNESDAY
W E E K 18	**AEROBICS** • Walk 3 min. at RPE <12; 17 min. at RPE = 12–13 (see Options 1). • Stationary cycle (dual-action) 20 min. at RPE = 12–13; 3 min. at RPE <12 (see Options 1). **STRENGTHENING** • 1 set of 12 reps of 9 exercises + 20 sit-ups. Use same weight/resistance; keep RPE <12. • 1 set of 12 reps of 9 exercises + 20 sit-ups. Use same weight/resistance; keep RPE = 12–15. **CONNORS COUNT = 19**	**AEROBICS** • Walk 3 min. at RPE <12; 40 min. at RPE = 12–13; 3 min. at RPE <12 (see Options 1). **CONNORS COUNT = 16**	**AEROBICS** • Walk 3 min. at RPE <12; 17 min. at RPE = 12–13 (see Options 1). • Stationary cycle (dual-action) 20 min. at RPE = 12–13; 3 min. at RPE <12 (see Options 1). **CONNORS COUNT = 17**

COMMENTS

• You are on your way to earning 100 points. Keep it up!

THURSDAY	FRIDAY	SATURDAY	SUNDAY

FRIDAY

AEROBICS
- Walk 3 min. at RPE <12; 17 min. at RPE = 12–13 (see Options 1).
- Stationary cycle (dual-action) 20 min. at RPE = 12–13; 3 min. at RPE <12 (see Options 1).

STRENGTHENING
- 1 set of 12 reps of 9 exercises + 20 sit-ups. Use same weight/resistance; keep RPE <12.
- 1 set of 12 reps of 9 exercises + 20 sit-ups. Use same weight/resistance; keep RPE = 12–15.

CONNORS COUNT = 19

SATURDAY

AEROBICS
- Walk 3 min. at RPE <12; 40 min. at RPE = 12–13; 3 min. at RPE <12 (see Options 1).

CONNORS COUNT = 16

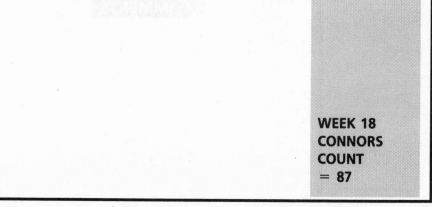

WEEK 18 CONNORS COUNT = 87

	MONDAY	TUESDAY	WEDNESDAY
W E E K 19	**AEROBICS** • Walk 3 min. at RPE <12; 20 min. at RPE = 12–13 (see Options 1). • Stationary cycle (dual-action) 20 min. at RPE = 12–13; 3 min. at RPE <12 (see Options 1). **STRENGTHENING** • 1 set of 12 reps of 9 exercises + 20 sit-ups. Use same weight/resistance; keep RPE <12. • 1 set of 12 reps of 9 exercises + 20 sit-ups. Use same weight/resistance; keep RPE = 12–15. **CONNORS COUNT = 20**	**AEROBICS** • Walk 3 min. at RPE <12; 45 min. at RPE = 12–13; 3 min. at RPE <12 (see Options 1). **CONNORS COUNT = 17**	**AEROBICS** • Walk 3 min. at RPE <12; 20 min. at RPE = 12–13 (see Options 1). • Stationary cycle (dual-action) 20 min. at RPE = 12–13; 3 min. at RPE <12 (see Options 1). **CONNORS COUNT = 18**

COMMENTS

• Great! You're almost there.

THURSDAY	FRIDAY	SATURDAY	SUNDAY
	AEROBICS • Walk 3 min. at RPE <12; 20 min. at RPE = 12–13 (see Options 1). • Stationary cycle (dual-action) 20 min. at RPE = 12–13; 3 min. at RPE <12 (see Options 1). **STRENGTHENING** • 1 set of 12 reps of 9 exercises + 20 sit-ups. Use same weight/resistance; keep RPE <12. • 1 set of 12 reps of 9 exercises + 20 sit-ups. Use same weight/resistance; keep RPE = 12–15. CONNORS COUNT = 20	**AEROBICS** • Walk 3 min. at RPE <12; 45 min. at RPE = 12–13; 3 min. at RPE <12 (see Options 1). CONNORS COUNT = 17	

**WEEK 19
CONNORS
COUNT
= 92**

	MONDAY	TUESDAY	WEDNESDAY
W E E K 20 A N D F O R E V E R	**AEROBICS** • Walk 3 min. at RPE <12; 20 min. at RPE = 12–13 (see Options 1). • Stationary cycle (dual-action) 20 min. at RPE = 12–13; 3 min. at RPE <12 (see Options 1). **STRENGTHENING** • 1 set of 12 reps of 9 exercises + 20 sit-ups. Use same weight/resistance; keep RPE <12. • 1 set of 12 reps of 9 exercises + 20 sit-ups. Use same weight/resistance; keep RPE = 12–15. **CONNORS COUNT = 20**	**AEROBICS** • Walk 3 min. at RPE <12; 54 min. at RPE = 12–13; 3 min. at RPE <12 (see Options 1). **CONNORS COUNT = 21**	**AEROBICS** • Walk 3 min. at RPE <12; 20 min. at RPE = 12–13 (see Options 1). • Stationary cycle (dual-action) 20 min. at RPE = 12–13; 3 min. at RPE <12 (see Options 1). **CONNORS COUNT = 18**

COMMENTS

• I'm proud of you! You are now performing an optimal amount of exercise from a health-related fitness standpoint. From here on out it's a question of maintenance. Congratulations.

THURSDAY	FRIDAY	SATURDAY	SUNDAY
	AEROBICS • Walk 3 min. at RPE <12; 20 min. at RPE = 12–13 (see Options 1). • Stationary cycle (dual-action) 20 min. at RPE = 12–13; 3 min. at RPE <12 (see Options 1). **STRENGTHENING** • 1 set of 12 reps of 9 exercises + 20 sit-ups. Use same weight/resistance; keep RPE <12. • 1 set of 12 reps of 9 exercises + 20 sit-ups. Use same weight/resistance; keep RPE = 12–15. CONNORS COUNT = 20	**AEROBICS** • Walk 3 min. at RPE <12; 54 min. at RPE = 12–13; 3 min. at RPE <12 (see Options 1). CONNORS COUNT = 21	

**WEEK 20
CONNORS
COUNT
= 100**

Program B

	MONDAY	TUESDAY	WEDNESDAY
W E E K 1	AEROBICS • Walk 15 min. at RPE <12; 5 min. at RPE = 12–13 (see Options 1). • Stationary cycle (dual-action) 7 min. at RPE <12 (see Options 1).		AEROBICS • Walk 13 min. at RPE <12; 7 min at RPE = 12–13 (see Options 1). • Stationary cycle (dual-action) 10 min. at RPE <12 (see Options 1).
	CONNORS COUNT = 6		CONNORS COUNT = 7

COMMENTS

• Way to go! During the course of the next 16 weeks I'm going to show you how to take your health and fitness to a new level. But keep in mind that even though you are already accustomed to regular exercise, I still want you to progress gradually.

• During the first two weeks I want you to start getting tuned in to your body with the use of the Borg Scale.

THURSDAY	FRIDAY	SATURDAY	SUNDAY

	AEROBICS
	  • Walk 10 min.
	at RPE <12; 10
	min. at RPE =
	12–13 (see Op-
	tions 1).
	  • Stationary
	cycle (dual-
	action) 12 min.
	at RPE <12 (see
	Options 1).		

	CONNORS COUNT = 8		

  • I also want you to get accustomed to a second aerobic activity—if
stationary cycling is not to your liking, select one of the other options.
  • Remember to stretch after each workout.

WEEK 1
CONNORS
COUNT
= 21

	MONDAY	**TUESDAY**	**WEDNESDAY**
W E E K 2	AEROBICS • Walk 7 min. at RPE <12; 13 min. at RPE = 12–13 (see Options 1). • Stationary cycle (dual-action) 15 min. at RPE <12 (see Options 1). STRENGTHENING • 1 set of 8 reps of 10 exercises. Select weight/resistance so that RPE <12.		AEROBICS • Walk 5 min. at RPE <12; 15 min. at RPE = 12–13 (see Options 1). • Stationary cycle (dual-action) 17 min. at RPE <12 (see Options 1).
	CONNORS COUNT = 10		CONNORS COUNT = 10

COMMENTS

• You may feel a little sore after your first few muscle-strengthening sessions. Provided it is not too severe, this "delayed onset muscle soreness" is quite normal and should disappear completely within a week or two after starting any new exercise.

• If you don't work out in a gym, use my home muscle-strengthening program (see the photo insert).

AEROBICS
• Walk 3 min. at RPE <12; 17 min. at RPE = 12–13 (see Options 1).
• Stationary cycle (dual-action) 20 min. at RPE <12 (see Options 1).

STRENGTHENING
• 1 set of 10 reps of 10 exercises. Use same weight/resistance; keep RPE <12.

CONNORS
COUNT
= 12

• If you rest for 60 seconds or less between each set of resistance exercises, you are performing what is known as "circuit training" and can count it toward the Connors Count. I suggest that you credit yourself with 0.5 minute of circuit training for each set of muscle-strengthening exercises.

**WEEK 2
CONNORS
COUNT
= 32**

	MONDAY	TUESDAY	WEDNESDAY
W E E K 3	**AEROBICS** • Stationary cycle (dual-action) 3 min. at RPE <12; 5 min. at RPE = 12–13; 12 min. at RPE <12 (see Options 1). **STRENGTHENING** • 1 set of 12 reps of 12 exercises. Use same weight/resistance; keep RPE <12.	**AEROBICS** • Walk 3 min. at RPE <12; walk 6 min. at RPE = 12–13; jog 1 min. at RPE = 12–13; walk 6 min. at RPE = 12–13; jog 1 min. at RPE = 12–13; walk 3 min. at RPE <12 (see Options 2).	
	CONNORS COUNT = 7	CONNORS COUNT = 7	

COMMENTS

• You're already earning more than the minimum weekly amount of aerobic exercise recommended by the American Heart Association.

• You are now adding an extra two workouts. To compensate for this and to give your body, especially your musculoskeletal system, a chance to adapt, I'm cutting back on your workouts on two of the other days (Monday and Friday) for the moment.

THURSDAY	FRIDAY	SATURDAY	SUNDAY
AEROBICS • Walk 3 min. at RPE <12; 17 min. at RPE = 12–13 (see Options 1). • Stationary cycle (dual-action) 7 min. at RPE = 12–13; 13 min. at RPE <12 (see Options 1).	**AEROBICS** • Stationary cycle (dual-action) 3 min. at RPE <12; 10 min. at RPE = 12–13; 7 min. at RPE <12 (see Options 1). **STRENGTHENING** • 1 set of 8 reps of 9 exercises + 14 sit-ups. Increase weight/resistance; keep RPE <12.	**AEROBICS** • Walk 3 min. at RPE <12; walk 5 min. at RPE = 12–13; jog 2 min. at RPE = 12–13; walk 5 min. at RPE = 12–13; jog 2 min. at RPE = 12–13; walk 3 min. at RPE <12 (see Options 2).	
CONNORS COUNT = 13	**CONNORS COUNT = 8**	**CONNORS COUNT = 7**	

• When you start jogging, do so at the same speed that you were walking—in other words, jog slowly. If your RPE exceeds a 13 while jogging, immediately slow down; you are jogging too fast.

• If you choose an option other than jogging that you are not familiar with, you may need to build up more gradually than I have suggested.

WEEK 3 CONNORS COUNT = 42

	MONDAY	**TUESDAY**	**WEDNESDAY**

W E E K 4

AEROBICS
• Stationary cycle (dual-action) 3 min. at RPE <12; 13 min. at RPE = 12–13; 4 min. at RPE <12 (see Options 1).

STRENGTHENING
• 1 set of 10 reps of 9 exercises + 16 sit-ups. Use same weight/resistance; keep RPE <12.
• 1 set of 8 reps of 10 exercises. Select weight/resistance so that RPE = 12–15.

CONNORS COUNT = 10

AEROBICS
• Walk 3 min. at RPE <12; walk 4 min. at RPE = 12–13; jog 3 min. at RPE = 12–13; walk 4 min. at RPE = 12–13; jog 3 min. at RPE = 12–13; walk 3 min. at RPE <12 (see Options 2).

CONNORS COUNT = 8

COMMENTS

• As you can see, I'm gradually increasing the time of each bout of jogging. Remember, slow down if your RPE goes above 13. If necessary, even slow down to a walk and alternate between shorter periods of walking and jogging than I have suggested.

• It's time to add a second set of muscle-strengthening exercises and to increase your RPE to a 12–15 for these (credit yourself with an extra 0.5 minute of circuit training per exercise when tallying your Connors Count).

THURSDAY	FRIDAY	SATURDAY	SUNDAY
AEROBICS • Walk 3 min. at RPE <12; 17 min. at RPE = 12–13 (see Options 1). • Stationary cycle (dual-action) 15 min. at RPE = 12–13; 5 min. at RPE <12 (see Options 1).	AEROBICS • Stationary cycle (dual-action) 3 min. at RPE <12; 17 min. at RPE = 12–13; 3 min. at RPE <12 (see Options 1). STRENGTHENING • 1 set of 12 reps of 9 exercises + 18 sit-ups. Use same weight/resistance; keep RPE <12. • 1 set of 8 reps of 10 exercises. Use same weight/resistance; keep RPE = 12–15.	AEROBICS • Walk 3 min. at RPE <12; walk 3 min. at RPE = 12–13; jog 4 min. at RPE = 12–13; walk 3 min. at RPE = 12–13; jog 4 min. at RPE = 12–13; walk 3 min. at RPE <12 (see Options 2).	
CONNORS COUNT = 15	CONNORS COUNT = 12	CONNORS COUNT = 8	

• Use the first set of each exercise as a warm-up set to reduce your risk of injury.

• You are now getting more than the minimum amount of strength training recommended by the American College of Sports Medicine.

WEEK 4 CONNORS COUNT = 53

	MONDAY	TUESDAY	WEDNESDAY
W E E K 5	**AEROBICS** • Stationary cycle (dual-action) 3 min. at RPE <12; 20 min. at RPE = 12–13; 3 min. at RPE <12 (see Options 1). **STRENGTHENING** • 1 set of 12 reps of 9 exercises + 20 sit-ups. Use same weight/resistance; keep RPE <12. • 1 set of 12 reps of 10 exercises. Use same weight/resistance; keep RPE = 12–15.	**AEROBICS** • Walk 3 min. at RPE <12; walk 2 min. at RPE = 12–13; jog 5 min. at RPE = 12–13; walk 2 min. at RPE = 12–13; jog 5 min. at RPE = 12–13; walk 3 min. at RPE <12 (see Options 2).	
	CONNORS COUNT = 13	**CONNORS COUNT = 9**	

COMMENTS

• You're doing fantastically! At the beginning of this week you will jog for 10 minutes in two 5-minute bouts. At the end I'm cutting your jogging down to a single 6-minute bout, which you will progressively lengthen over the next few weeks.

THURSDAY	FRIDAY	SATURDAY	SUNDAY
AEROBICS • Walk 3 min. at RPE <12; 17 min. at RPE = 12–13 (see Options 1). • Stationary cycle (dual-action) 17 min. at RPE = 12–13; 3 min. at RPE <12 (see Options 1).	AEROBICS • Stationary cycle (dual-action) 3 min. at RPE <12; 20 min. at RPE = 12–13; 3 min. at RPE <12 (see Options 1). STRENGTHENING • 1 set of 12 reps of 9 exercises + 20 sit-ups. Use same weight/resistance; keep RPE <12. • 1 set of 12 reps of 9 exercises + 14 sit-ups. Use same weight/resistance; keep RPE = 12–15.	AEROBICS • Walk 3 min. at RPE <12; jog 6 min. at RPE = 12–13; walk 8 min. at RPE = 12–13; walk 3 min. at RPE <12 (see Options 2).	
CONNORS COUNT = 15	CONNORS COUNT = 13	CONNORS COUNT = 8	

• The 3 minutes of aerobic exercise at an RPE <12 at the beginning and end of each aerobic workout are intended as a warm-up and cool-down; however, you still take credit for them when using the Connors Count.

WEEK 5 CONNORS COUNT = 58

	MONDAY	TUESDAY	WEDNESDAY

WEEK 6

MONDAY

AEROBICS
• Stationary cycle (dual-action) 3 min. at RPE <12; 22 min. at RPE = 12–13; 3 min. at RPE <12 (see Options 1).

STRENGTHENING
• 1 set of 12 reps of 9 exercises + 20 sit-ups. Use same weight/resistance; keep RPE <12.
• 1 set of 8 reps of 9 exercises + 16 sit-ups. Increase weight/resistance; keep RPE = 12–15.

CONNORS COUNT = 14

TUESDAY

AEROBICS
• Walk 3 min. at RPE <12; jog 8 min. at RPE = 12–13; walk 6 min. at RPE = 12–13; walk 3 min. at RPE <12 (see Options 2).

CONNORS COUNT = 8

COMMENTS

• You're back up to 10 minutes of jogging. But now you are doing it in a single bout rather than in two 5-minute bouts.
• It's time to increase the weight/resistance you are using during strength training. When doing so, remember to drop your number of repetitions back down to 8 and keep your RPE at 12–15. Because your

THURSDAY	FRIDAY	SATURDAY	SUNDAY
AEROBICS • Walk 3 min. at RPE <12; 17 min. at RPE = 12–13 (see Options 1). • Stationary cycle (dual-action) 17 min. at RPE = 12–13; 3 min. at RPE <12 (see Options 1).	**AEROBICS** • Stationary cycle (dual-action) 3 min. at RPE <12; 22 min. at RPE = 12–13; 3 min. at RPE <12 (see Options 1). **STRENGTHENING** • 1 set of 12 reps of 9 exercises + 20 sit-ups. Use same weight/resistance; keep RPE <12. • 1 set of 8 reps of 9 exercises + 18 sit-ups. Use same weight/resistance; keep RPE = 12–15.	**AEROBICS** • Walk 3 min. at RPE <12; jog 10 min. at RPE = 12–13; walk 4 min. at RPE = 12–13; walk 3 min. at RPE <12 (see Options 2).	
CONNORS COUNT = 15	CONNORS COUNT = 14	CONNORS COUNT = 9	

first set of each exercise is intended as a warm-up, you don't need to change the weight/resistance you are using for it—keep it fairly easy.

WEEK 6 CONNORS COUNT = 60

	MONDAY	TUESDAY	WEDNESDAY
W E E K 7	**AEROBICS** • Stationary cycle (dual-action) 3 min. at RPE <12; 24 min. at RPE = 12–13; 3 min. at RPE <12 (see Options 1). **STRENGTHENING** • 1 set of 12 reps of 9 exercises + 20 sit-ups. Use same weight/resistance; keep RPE <12. • 1 set of 10 reps of 9 exercises + 20 sit-ups. Use same weight/resistance; keep RPE = 12–15. CONNORS COUNT = 15	**AEROBICS** • Walk 3 min. at RPE <12; jog 12 min. at RPE = 12–13; walk 3 min. at RPE <12 (see Options 2). CONNORS COUNT = 8	

COMMENTS

• With all the attention I'm focusing on building up the length of time you are able to jog, don't forget to stretch after each workout. Continue to perform 2 to 3 gentle repetitions of the stretching exercises shown in the photo insert.

THURSDAY	FRIDAY	SATURDAY	SUNDAY
AEROBICS • Walk 3 min. at RPE <12; 17 min. at RPE = 12–13 (see Options 1). • Stationary cycle (dual-action) 17 min. at RPE = 12–13; 3 min. at RPE <12 (see Options 1).	**AEROBICS** • Stationary cycle (dual-action) 3 min. at RPE <12; 24 min. at RPE = 12–13; 3 min. at RPE <12 (see Options 1). **STRENGTHENING** • 1 set of 12 reps of 9 exercises + 20 sit-ups. Use same weight/resistance; keep RPE <12. • 1 set of 10 reps of 9 exercises + 20 sit-ups. Use same weight/resistance; keep RPE = 12–15.	**AEROBICS** • Walk 3 min. at RPE <12; jog 14 min. at RPE = 12–13; walk 3 min. at RPE = 12–13; walk 3 min. at RPE <12 (see Options 2).	
CONNORS COUNT = 15	**CONNORS COUNT = 15**	**CONNORS COUNT = 10**	

WEEK 7 CONNORS COUNT = 63

	MONDAY	TUESDAY	WEDNESDAY

W E E K 8

MONDAY

AEROBICS
• Stationary cycle (dual-action) 3 min. at RPE <12; 24 min. at RPE = 12–13; 3 min. at RPE <12 (see Options 1).

STRENGTHENING
• 1 set of 12 reps of 9 exercises + 20 sit-ups. Use same weight/resistance; keep RPE <12.
• 1 set of 12 reps of 9 exercises + 20 sit-ups. Use same weight/resistance; keep RPE = 12–15.

CONNORS COUNT = 15

TUESDAY

AEROBICS
• Walk 3 min. at RPE <12; jog 17 min. at RPE = 12–13; walk 3 min. at RPE <12 (see Options 2).

CONNORS COUNT = 11

WEDNESDAY

COMMENTS

• Keep up the great work! You are already jogging for 20 minutes at a time. Not many adults can do this without exhausting themselves.

THURSDAY	FRIDAY	SATURDAY	SUNDAY
AEROBICS • Walk 3 min. at RPE <12; 17 min. at RPE = 12–13 (see Options 1). • Stationary cycle (dual-action) 17 min. at RPE = 12–13; 3 min. at RPE <12 (see Options 1).	AEROBICS • Stationary cycle (dual-action) 3 min. at RPE <12; 24 min. at RPE = 12–13; 3 min. at RPE <12 (see Options 1). STRENGTHENING • 1 set of 12 reps of 9 exercises + 20 sit-ups. Use same weight/resistance; keep RPE <12. • 1 set of 12 reps of 9 exercises + 20 sit-ups. Use same weight/resistance; keep RPE = 12–15.	AEROBICS • Walk 3 min. at RPE <12; jog 20 min. at RPE = 12–13; walk 3 min. at RPE <12 (see Options 2).	
CONNORS COUNT = 15	CONNORS COUNT = 15	CONNORS COUNT = 13	

WEEK 8 CONNORS COUNT = 69

	MONDAY	TUESDAY	WEDNESDAY

W E E K 9

MONDAY

AEROBICS
• Stationary cycle (dual-action) 3 min. at RPE <12; 20 min. at RPE = 12–13 (see Options 1).
• Jump rope/march in place 30 sec. at RPE = 14–15; walk 2 min. at RPE <12; jump rope/march in place 30 sec. at RPE = 13–15; walk 3 min. at RPE <12 (see Options 2).

STRENGTHENING
• 1 set of 12 reps of 9 exercises + 20 sit-ups. Use same weight/resistance; keep RPE <12.
• 1 set of 8 reps of 9 exercises + 20 sit-ups. Increase weight/resistance; keep RPE = 12–15.

CONNORS COUNT = 14

TUESDAY

AEROBICS
• Walk 3 min. at RPE <12; jog 22 min. at RPE = 12–13; walk 3 min. at RPE <12 (see Options 2).

CONNORS COUNT = 14

COMMENTS

• OK! You are now ready to include a third aerobic activity in your program, should you wish to. Jumping rope is my favorite and you may want to give it a try. Keep in mind it's a strenuous activity; you will probably have to exercise at an RPE of 14–15 if you've not performed this activity regularly in the past. If your RPE goes above 15, immediately stop jumping and march in place until you feel ready to continue again; keep

THURSDAY	FRIDAY	SATURDAY	SUNDAY
AEROBICS • Walk 3 min. at RPE <12; 17 min. at RPE = 12–13 (see Options 1). • Stationary cycle (dual-action) 17 min. at RPE = 12–13; 3 min. at RPE <12 (see Options 1).	**AEROBICS** • Stationary cycle (dual-action) 3 min. at RPE <12; 20 min. at RPE = 12–13 (see Options 1). • Jump rope/march in place 30 sec. at RPE = 14–15; walk 2 min. at RPE <12; jump rope/march in place 30 sec. at RPE = 14–15; walk 3 min. at RPE <12 (see Options 2). **STRENGTHENING** • 1 set of 12 reps of 9 exercises + 20 sit-ups. Use same weight/resistance; keep RPE <12. • 1 set of 8 reps of 9 exercises + 20 sit-ups. Increase weight/resistance; keep RPE = 12–15.	**AEROBICS** • Walk 3 min. at RPE <12; jog 22 min. at RPE = 12–13; walk 3 min. at RPE <12 (see Options 2).	
CONNORS COUNT = 15	**CONNORS COUNT = 14**	**CONNORS COUNT = 14**	

repeating this process until you complete the time I have recommended (when doing this, credit yourself with the same number of points as if you had jumped without interruption). It's time to increase the weight/resistance you are using during strength training.

WEEK 9 CONNORS COUNT = 71

	MONDAY	**TUESDAY**	**WEDNESDAY**
W **E** **E** **K** **10**	**AEROBICS** • Stationary cycle (dual-action) 3 min. at RPE <12; 22 min. at RPE = 12–13 (see Options 1). • Jump rope/march in place 1 min. at RPE = 14–15; walk 2 min. at RPE <12; jump rope/march in place 1 min. at RPE = 14–15; walk 3 min. at RPE <12 (see Options 2). **STRENGTHENING** • 1 set of 12 reps of 9 exercises + 20 sit-ups. Use same weight/resistance; keep RPE <12. • 1 set of 10 reps of 9 exercises + 20 sit-ups. Use same weight/resistance; keep RPE = 12–15. **CONNORS COUNT = 16**	**AEROBICS** • Walk 3 min. at RPE <12; jog 25 min. at RPE = 12–13; walk 3 min. at RPE <12 (see Options 2). **CONNORS COUNT = 16**	

COMMENTS

• You are over the 75-point mark—fantastic!
• One minute of jumping rope can feel like a pretty long time if you're not used to it. Don't hesitate to stop jumping and start marching in place if you can't complete the entire minute without your RPE exceeding a 15. As you become fitter and more proficient at jumping rope, you won't need to stop as much. However, I will still recommend that you do

THURSDAY	FRIDAY	SATURDAY	SUNDAY
AEROBICS • Walk 3 min. at RPE <12; 17 min. at RPE = 12–13 (see Options 1). • Stationary cycle (dual-action) 17 min. at RPE = 12–13; 3 min. at RPE <12 (see Options 1).	AEROBICS • Stationary cycle (dual-action) 3 min. at RPE <12; 22 min. at RPE = 12–13 (see Options 1). • Jump rope/march in place 1 min. at RPE = 14–15; walk 2 min. at RPE <12; jump rope/march in place 1 min. at RPE = 14–15; walk 3 min. at RPE <12 (see Options 2). STRENGTHENING • 1 set of 12 reps of 9 exercises + 20 sit-ups. Use same weight/resistance; keep RPE <12. • 1 set of 10 reps of 9 exercises + 20 sit-ups. Use same weight/resistance; keep RPE = 12–15.	AEROBICS • Walk 3 min. at RPE <12; jog 25 min. at RPE = 12–13; walk 3 min. at RPE <12 (see Options 2).	
CONNORS COUNT = 15	CONNORS COUNT = 16	CONNORS COUNT = 16	

your rope jumping in several rounds—it's what I do during my workouts.
• Jumping rope is a fairly high-impact activity. If you start experiencing pain or discomfort in your muscles, bones, or joints, you need to cut back or switch to another activity.

WEEK 10 CONNORS COUNT = 79

	MONDAY	**TUESDAY**	**WEDNESDAY**
W E E K 11	AEROBICS • Stationary cycle (dual-action) 3 min. at RPE <12; 25 min. at RPE = 12–13 (see Options 1). • Jump rope/march in place 1.5 min. at RPE = 14–15; walk 2 min. at RPE <12; jump rope/march in place 1.5 min. at RPE = 14–15; walk 3 min. at RPE <12 (see Options 2). STRENGTHENING • 1 set of 12 reps of 9 exercises + 20 sit-ups. Use same weight/resistance; keep RPE <12. • 1 set of 12 reps of 9 exercises + 20 sit-ups. Use same weight/resistance; keep RPE = 12–15. CONNORS COUNT = 18	AEROBICS • Walk 3 min. at RPE <12; jog 20 min. at RPE = 12–13; walk 3 min. at RPE <12 (see Options 2). CONNORS COUNT = 13	

COMMENTS

• You should be starting to get the hang of jumping rope. Now I want you to start jogging on an extra day each week. To accomplish this without overstressing your musculoskeletal system, I'm cutting back slightly on

THURSDAY	FRIDAY	SATURDAY	SUNDAY
AEROBICS • Walk 3 min. at RPE <12; jog 15 min. at RPE = 12–13 (see Options 2). • Stationary cycle (dual-action) 17 min. at RPE = 12–13; 3 min. at RPE <12 (see Options 1).	**AEROBICS** • Stationary cycle (dual-action) 3 min. at RPE <12; 25 min. at RPE = 12–13 (see Options 1). • Jump rope/march in place 1.5 min. at RPE = 14–15; walk 2 min. at RPE <12; jump rope/march in place 1.5 min. at RPE = 14–15; walk 3 min. at RPE <12 (see Options 2). **STRENGTHENING** • 1 set of 12 reps of 9 exercises + 20 sit-ups. Use same weight/resistance; keep RPE <12. • 1 set of 12 reps of 9 exercises + 20 sit-ups. Use same weight/resistance; keep RPE = 12–15.	**AEROBICS** • Walk 3 min. at RPE <12; jog 20 min. at RPE = 12–13; walk 3 min. at RPE <12 (see Options 2).	
CONNORS COUNT = 18	CONNORS COUNT = 18	CONNORS COUNT = 13	

your Tuesday and Saturday workouts and asking you to jog instead of walk during Thursday's workout.

WEEK 11 CONNORS COUNT = 80

	MONDAY	TUESDAY	WEDNESDAY

WEEK 12

MONDAY

AEROBICS
• Stationary cycle (dual-action) 3 min. at RPE <12; 25 min. at RPE = 12–13 (see Options 1).
• Jump rope/ march in place 2 min. at RPE = 14–15; walk 2 min. at RPE <12; jump rope/ march in place 2 min. at RPE = 14–15; walk 3 min. at RPE <12 (see Options 2).

STRENGTHENING
• 1 set of 12 reps of 9 exercises + 20 sit-ups. Use same weight/resistance; keep RPE <12.
• 1 set of 8 reps of 9 exercises + 20 sit-ups. Increase weight/resistance; keep RPE = 12–15.

CONNORS COUNT = 19

TUESDAY

AEROBICS
• Walk 3 min. at RPE <12; jog 20 min. at RPE = 12–13; walk 3 min. at RPE <12 (see Options 2).

CONNORS COUNT = 13

COMMENTS

• It's time to increase the amount of weight/resistance you are using for your muscle-strengthening exercises.
• Although I haven't included it in your program, this is the time to

THURSDAY	FRIDAY	SATURDAY	SUNDAY

AEROBICS
• Walk 3 min. at RPE <12; jog 17 min. at RPE = 12–13 (see Options 2).
• Stationary cycle (dual-action) 17 min. at RPE = 12–13; 3 min. at RPE <12 (see Options 1).

AEROBICS
• Stationary cycle (dual-action) 3 min. at RPE <12; 25 min. at RPE = 12–13 (see Options 1).
• Jump rope/ march in place 2 min. at RPE = 14–15; walk 2 min. at RPE <12; jump rope/ march in place 2 min. at RPE = 14–15; walk 3 min. at RPE <12 (see Options 2).

STRENGTHENING
• 1 set of 12 reps of 9 exercises + 20 sit-ups. Use same weight/resistance; keep RPE <12.
• 1 set of 8 reps of 9 exercises + 20 sit-ups. Use same weight/resistance; keep RPE = 12–15.

AEROBICS
• Walk 3 min. at RPE <12; jog 20 min. at RPE = 12–13; walk 3 min. at RPE <12 (see Options 2).

CONNORS COUNT = 20

CONNORS COUNT = 19

CONNORS COUNT = 13

consider adding a third set of each muscle-strengthening exercise to your routine; do so if you have the time and if improving your body is high on the priority list of reasons why you started working out.

**WEEK 12
CONNORS
COUNT
= 84**

	MONDAY	TUESDAY	WEDNESDAY
W E E K 13	**AEROBICS** • Stationary cycle (dual-action) 3 min. at RPE <12; 22 min. at RPE = 12–13 (see Options 1). • Jump rope/march in place 2 min. at RPE = 14–15; walk 2 min. at RPE <12; jump rope/march in place 2 min. at RPE = 14–15; walk 2 min. at RPE <12; jump rope/march in place 1 min. at RPE = 14–15; walk 3 min. at RPE <12 (see Options 2). **STRENGTHENING** • 1 set of 12 reps of 9 exercises + 20 sit-ups. Use same weight/resistance; keep RPE < 12. • 1 set of 10 reps of 9 exercises + 20 sit-ups. Use same weight/resistance; keep RPE = 12–15. **CONNORS COUNT = 19**	**AEROBICS** • Walk 3 min. at RPE <12; jog 22 min. at RPE = 12–13; walk 3 min. at RPE <12 (see Options 2). **CONNORS COUNT = 14**	

COMMENTS

• I'm adding a third round of jumping rope to your Monday and Friday workouts. This will have a dramatic impact on your functional fitness

THURSDAY	FRIDAY	SATURDAY	SUNDAY

AEROBICS
- Walk 3 min. at RPE <12; jog 17 min. at RPE = 12–13 (see Options 2).
- Stationary cycle (dual-action) 17 min. at RPE = 12–13; 3 min at RPE <12 (see Options 1).

AEROBICS
- Stationary cycle (dual-action) 3 min. at RPE <12; 22 min. at RPE = 12–13 (see Options 1).
- Jump rope/march in place 2 min. at RPE = 14–15; walk 2 min. at RPE <12; jump rope/march in place 2 min. at RPE = 14–15; walk 2 min. at RPE <12; jump rope/march in place 1 min. at RPE = 14–15; walk 3 min. at RPE <12 (see Options 2).

STRENGTHENING
- 1 set of 12 reps of 9 exercises + 20 sit-ups. Use same weight/resistance; keep RPE <12.
- 1 set of 10 reps of 9 exercises + 20 sit-ups. Use same weight/resistance; keep RPE = 12–15.

AEROBICS
- Walk 3 min. at RPE <12; jog 22 min. at RPE = 12–13; walk 3 min. at RPE <12 (see Options 2).

CONNORS COUNT = 20

CONNORS COUNT = 19

CONNORS COUNT = 14

level. Because your time is precious, I'm cutting back a bit on your cycling on these days.

WEEK 13 CONNORS COUNT = 86

	MONDAY	TUESDAY	WEDNESDAY

WEEK 14

MONDAY

AEROBICS
• Stationary cycle (dual-action) 3 min. at RPE <12; 22 min. at RPE = 12–13 (see Options 1).
• Jump rope/march in place 2.5 min. at RPE = 14–15; walk 2 min. at RPE <12; jump rope/march in place 2.5 min. at RPE = 14–15; walk 2 min. at RPE <12; jump rope/march in place 2 min. at RPE = 14–15; walk 3 min. at RPE <12 (see Options 2).

STRENGTHENING
• 1 set of 12 reps of 9 exercises + 20 sit-ups. Use same weight/resistance; keep RPE <12.
• 1 set of 12 reps of 9 exercises + 20 sit-ups. Use same weight/resistance; keep RPE = 12–15.

CONNORS COUNT = 20

TUESDAY

AEROBICS
• Walk 3 min. at RPE <12; jog 25 min. at RPE = 12–13; walk 3 min. at RPE <12 (see Options 2).

CONNORS COUNT = 16

COMMENTS

• You're almost there—dont't count yourself out!

THURSDAY	FRIDAY	SATURDAY	SUNDAY
AEROBICS • Walk 3 min. at RPE <12; jog 17 min. at RPE = 12–13 (see Options 2). • Stationary cycle (dual-action) 17 min. at RPE = 12–13; 3 min. at RPE <12 (see Options 1).	**AEROBICS** • Stationary cycle (dual-action) 3 min. at RPE <12; 22 min. at RPE = 12–13 (see Options 1). • Jump rope/march in place 2.5 min. at 5 RPE = 14–15; walk 2 min. at RPE <12; jump rope/march in place 2.5 min at RPE = 14–15; walk 2 min. at RPE <12; jump rope/march in place 2 min. at RPE = 14–15; walk 3 min. at RPE <12 (see Options 2). **STRENGTHENING** • 1 set of 12 reps of 9 exercises + 20 sit-ups. Use same weight/resistance; keep RPE <12. • 1 set of 12 reps of 9 exercises + 20 sit-ups. Use same weight/resistance; keep RPE = 12–15.	**AEROBICS** • Walk 3 min. at RPE <12; jog 25 min. at RPE = 12–13; walk 3 min. at RPE <12 (see Options 2).	
CONNORS COUNT = 20	CONNORS COUNT = 20	CONNORS COUNT = 16	

WEEK 14 CONNORS COUNT = 92

	MONDAY	TUESDAY	WEDNESDAY

W E E K 15

MONDAY

AEROBICS
- Stationary cycle (dual-action) 3 min. at RPE <12; 22 min. at RPE = 12–13 (see Options 1).
- Jump rope/ march in place 3 min. at RPE = 14–15; walk 2 min. at RPE <12; jump rope/march in place 2 min. at RPE = 14–15; walk 3 min. at RPE <12 (see Options 2).

STRENGTHENING
- 1 set of 12 reps of 9 exercises + 20 sit-ups. Use same weight/resistance; keep RPE = 12–15.
- 1 set of 12 reps of 9 exercises + 20 sit-ups. Use same weight/resistance; keep RPE = 12–15.

CONNORS COUNT = 21

TUESDAY

AEROBICS
- Walk 3 min. at RPE <12; jog 27 min. at RPE = 12–13; walk 3 min. at RPE <12 (see Options 2).

CONNORS COUNT = 17

WEDNESDAY

COMMENTS

- If improving your body is high on your priority list of reasons for exercising and you have the time, consider increasing the frequency of your muscle-strengthening workouts to three days per week.

THURSDAY	FRIDAY	SATURDAY	SUNDAY
AEROBICS • Walk 3 min. at RPE <12; jog 17 min. at RPE = 12–13 (see Options 2). • Stationary cycle (dual-action) 17 min. at RPE = 12–13; 3 min. at RPE <12 (see Options 1).	AEROBICS • Stationary cycle (dual-action) 3 min. at RPE <12; 22 min. at RPE = 12–13 (see Options 1). • Jump rope/march in place 3 min. at RPE = 14–15; walk 2 min. at RPE <12; jump rope/march in place 3 min. at RPE = 14–15; walk 2 min. at RPE <12 jump rope/march in place 2 min. at RPE = 14–15; walk 3 min. at RPE <12 (see Options 2). STRENGTHENING • 1 set of 12 reps of 9 exercises + 20 sit-ups. Use same weight/resistance; keep RPE <12. • 1 set of 12 reps of 9 exercises + 20 sit-ups. Use same weight/resistance; keep RPE = 12–15.	AEROBICS • Walk 3 min. at RPE <12; jog 27 min. at RPE = 12–13; walk 3 min. at RPE <12 (see Options 2).	
CONNORS COUNT = 20	CONNORS COUNT = 21	CONNORS COUNT = 17	

**WEEK 15
CONNORS
COUNT
= 96**

	MONDAY	TUESDAY	WEDNESDAY

WEEK 16 AND FOREVER

MONDAY

AEROBICS
- Stationary cycle (dual-action) 3 min. at RPE <12; 22 min. at RPE = 12–13 (see Options 1).
- Jump rope/march in place 3 min. at RPE = 14–15; walk 2 min. at RPE <12; jump rope/march in place 3 min. at RPE = 14–15; walk 2 min. at RPE <12; jump rope/march in place 3 min. at RPE = 14–15; walk 3 min. at RPE <12 (see Options 2).

STRENGTHENING
- 1 set of 12 reps of 9 exercises + 20 sit-ups. Use same weight/resistance; keep RPE <12.
- 1 set of 12 reps of 9 exercises + 20 sit-ups. Use same weight/resistance; keep RPE = 12–15.

CONNORS COUNT = 21

TUESDAY

AEROBICS
- Walk 3 min. at RPE <12; jog 30 min. at RPE = 12–13; walk 3 min. at RPE <12 (see Options 2).

CONNORS COUNT = 19

COMMENTS

- I'm proud of you! You are now performing the maximum amount of exercise needed from a health-related fitness standpoint. There is no

THURSDAY	FRIDAY	SATURDAY	SUNDAY
AEROBICS • Walk 3 min. at RPE <12; jog 17 min. at RPE = 12–13 (see Options 2). • Stationary cycle (dual-action) 17 min. at RPE = 12–13; 3 min. at RPE <12 (see Options 1).	**AEROBICS** • Stationary cycle (dual-action) 3 min. at RPE <12; 22 min. at RPE = 12–13 (see Options 1). • Jump rope/march in place 3 min. at RPE = 14–15; walk 2 min. at RPE <12; jump rope/march in place 3 min. at RPE = 14–15; walk 2 min. at RPE <12; jump rope/march in place 3 min. at RPE = 14–15; walk 3 min. at RPE <12 (see Options 2). **STRENGTHENING** • 1 set of 12 reps of 9 exercises + 20 sit-ups. Use same weight/resistance; keep RPE <12. • 1 set of 12 reps of 9 exercises + 20 sit-ups. Use same weight/resistance; keep RPE = 12–15.	**AEROBICS** • Walk 3 min. at RPE <12; jog 30 min. at RPE = 12–13; walk 3 min. at RPE <12 (see Options 2).	
CONNORS COUNT = 20	CONNORS COUNT = 21	CONNORS COUNT = 19	

reason to do more than this. From here on out, perform this same amount of exercise each week for maintenance. Congratulations!

**WEEK 16
CONNORS
COUNT
= 100**

THE CONNORS COUNT® INDEX

Activity	Intensity*		
	Low (RPE < 12)	**Moderate** (RPE = 12–13)	**High** (RPE > 13)
Aerobic dancing	Chart E	Chart G	Chart J
Aerobic dancing (bench/step training)	Chart E	Chart I	Chart M
Alpine skiing	Chart E	Chart G	Chart I
Aqua-aerobics	Chart E	Chart G	Chart J
Backpacking	Chart G	Chart I	Chart K
Badminton	Chart C	Chart G	Chart J
Ballet	Chart F	Chart G	Chart I
Ball games	Chart C	Chart E	Chart F
Ball hockey	Chart C	Chart E	Chart F
Ballroom dancing	Chart C	Chart E	Chart F
Baseball	Chart C	Chart E	Chart F
Basketball	Chart G	Chart I	Chart L
Bicycling	Chart C	Chart H	Chart K
Bowling	Chart A	Chart B	Chart C
Boxing	Chart G	Chart J	Chart M
Canoeing	Chart C	Chart E	Chart G
Catch (ball)	Chart C	Chart E	Chart F
Circuit weight training	Chart C	Chart F	Chart H
Cricket	Chart C	Chart E	Chart F
Croquet	Chart A	Chart B	Chart C
Cross-country skiing	Chart F	Chart J	Chart N
Curling	Chart E	Chart F	Chart G
Disco and popular dancing	Chart C	Chart F	Chart H
Exercise classes	Chart E	Chart G	Chart J
Fencing	Chart F	Chart H	Chart K
Figure skating	Chart E	Chart G	Chart K
Folk dancing	Chart C	Chart F	Chart H

| Activity | Intensity* | | |
	Low (RPE < 12)	Moderate (RPE = 12–13)	High (RPE > 13)
Football (American)	Chart F	Chart G	Chart H
Football (touch)	Chart F	Chart G	Chart I
Frisbee	Chart C	Chart E	Chart F
Gardening (digging, raking, weeding)	Chart C	Chart E	Chart F
Golf	Chart B	Chart D	Chart F
Gymnastics	Chart F	Chart H	Chart K
Handball (4-wall)	Chart G	Chart I	Chart L
Heavy housework (carpentry, painting, washing floors, washing windows)	Chart C	Chart D	Chart F
Hiking	Chart C	Chart G	Chart I
Home calisthenics	Chart C	Chart F	Chart I
Hunting	Chart C	Chart F	Chart H
Ice hockey	Chart G	Chart I	Chart K
Jogging	Chart H	Chart K	Chart M
Judo	Chart G	Chart I	Chart M
Jumping rope	Chart H	Chart K	Chart M
Karate	Chart F	Chart I	Chart M
Kayaking	Chart G	Chart I	Chart L
Lacrosse	Chart G	Chart I	Chart K
Modern dancing	Chart F	Chart G	Chart I
Mountaineering	Chart H	Chart I	Chart K
Mowing lawn (push mower)	Chart C	Chart E	Chart F
Orienteering	Chart I	Chart K	Chart M
Racquetball	Chart G	Chart J	Chart M
Rebounding	Chart D	Chart F	Chart G
Roller skating	Chart F	Chart H	Chart I
Rowing	Chart H	Chart K	Chart N

Activity	Intensity*		
	Low (RPE < 12)	**Moderate** (RPE = 12–13)	**High** (RPE > 13)
Rugby	Chart G	Chart I	Chart L
Sailing (small boat)	Chart C	Chart E	Chart G
Scuba diving	Chart E	Chart F	Chart G
Sculling	Chart E	Chart G	Chart K
Skateboarding	Chart F	Chart H	Chart I
Skating (ice)	Chart E	Chart H	Chart N
Snorkeling	Chart E	Chart F	Chart G
Snowmobiling	Chart C	Chart D	Chart F
Snow shoveling	Chart E	Chart G	Chart I
Soccer	Chart F	Chart H	Chart L
Softball	Chart C	Chart E	Chart F
Square dancing	Chart C	Chart F	Chart H
Squash	Chart G	Chart J	Chart M
Stair climbing/stepping	Chart E	Chart H	Chart L
Stationary cycling (legs only)	Chart C	Chart H	Chart K
Stationary cycling (arms only)	Chart B	Chart E	Chart H
Stationary cycling (dual-action)	Chart D	Chart I	Chart M
Swimming (beach)	Chart A	Chart C	Chart E
Swimming (pool)	Chart C	Chart F	Chart J
Synchronized swimming	Chart E	Chart G	Chart I
Table tennis	Chart E	Chart G	Chart J
Tag games	Chart C	Chart E	Chart F
Tennis	Chart E	Chart H	Chart K
Tobogganing	Chart F	Chart G	Chart H
Trail biking	Chart E	Chart F	Chart H
Volleyball	Chart F	Chart G	Chart I
Walking	Chart C	Chart G	Chart K

	Intensity*		
Activity	Low (RPE < 12)	Moderate (RPE = 12–13)	High (RPE > 13)
Walking (treadmill, with incline)	Chart E	Chart I	Chart L
Walking (upstairs)	Chart E	Chart H	Chart L
Walk-jog	Chart F	Chart I	Chart L
Waterskiing	Chart F	Chart H	Chart J
Windsurfing	Chart E	Chart F	Chart H
Woodcutting	Chart E	Chart F	Chart H
Wrestling	Chart G	Chart J	Chart M

*Low intensity (RPE of less than 12) generally results in minimal perspiration and only a slight increase in breathing above normal. Moderate intensity (RPE of 12 to 13) results in definite perspiration and above normal breathing. High intensity (RPE of more than 13) results in heavy perspiration and breathing.

THE CONNORS COUNT™ CHART A

Time (minutes)	Points	Time (minutes)	Points	Time (minutes)	Points	Time (minutes)	Points
1	0.1	16	1.0	31	1.9	46	2.8
2	0.1	17	1.0	32	1.9	47	2.8
3	0.2	18	1.1	33	2.0	48	2.9
4	0.2	19	1.1	34	2.0	49	2.9
5	0.3	20	1.2	35	2.1	50	3.0
6	0.4	21	1.3	36	2.2	51	3.1
7	0.4	22	1.3	37	2.2	52	3.1
8	0.5	23	1.4	38	2.3	53	3.2
9	0.5	24	1.4	39	2.3	54	3.2
10	0.6	25	1.5	40	2.4	55	3.3
11	0.7	26	1.6	41	2.5	56	3.4
12	0.7	27	1.6	42	2.5	57	3.4
13	0.8	28	1.7	43	2.6	58	3.5
14	0.8	29	1.7	44	2.6	59	3.5
15	0.9	30	1.8	45	2.7	60	3.6

THE CONNORS COUNT® CHART B

Time (minutes)	Points	Time (minutes)	Points	Time (minutes)	Points	Time (minutes)	Points
1	0.2	16	2.4	31	4.7	46	6.9
2	0.3	17	2.6	32	4.8	47	7.1
3	0.5	18	2.7	33	5.0	48	7.2
4	0.6	19	2.9	34	5.1	49	7.4
5	0.8	20	3.0	35	5.3	50	7.5
6	0.9	21	3.2	36	5.4	51	7.7
7	1.1	22	3.3	37	5.6	52	7.8
8	1.2	23	3.5	38	5.7	53	8.0
9	1.4	24	3.6	39	5.9	54	8.1
10	1.5	25	3.8	40	6.0	55	8.3
11	1.7	26	3.9	41	6.2	56	8.4
12	1.8	27	4.1	42	6.3	57	8.6
13	2.0	28	4.2	43	6.5	58	8.7
14	2.1	29	4.4	44	6.6	59	8.9
15	2.3	30	4.5	45	6.8	60	9.0

THE CONNORS COUNT® CHART C

Time (minutes)	Points	Time (minutes)	Points	Time (minutes)	Points	Time (minutes)	Points
1	0.2	16	2.9	31	5.6	46	8.3
2	0.4	17	3.1	32	5.8	47	8.5
3	0.5	18	3.2	33	5.9	48	8.6
4	0.7	19	3.4	34	6.1	49	8.8
5	0.9	20	3.6	35	6.3	50	9.0
6	1.1	21	3.8	36	6.5	51	9.2
7	1.3	22	4.0	37	6.7	52	9.4
8	1.4	23	4.1	38	6.8	53	9.5
9	1.6	24	4.3	39	7.0	54	9.7
10	1.8	25	4.5	40	7.2	55	9.9
11	2.0	26	4.7	41	7.4	56	10.1
12	2.2	27	4.9	42	7.6	57	10.3
13	2.3	28	5.0	43	7.7	58	10.4
14	2.5	29	5.2	44	7.9	59	10.6
15	2.7	30	5.4	45	8.1	60	10.8

THE CONNORS COUNT® CHART D

Time (minutes)	Points	Time (minutes)	Points	Time (minutes)	Points	Time (minutes)	Points
1	0.2	16	3.4	31	6.5	46	9.7
2	0.4	17	3.6	32	6.7	47	9.9
3	0.6	18	3.8	33	6.9	48	10.1
4	0.8	19	4.0	34	7.1	49	10.3
5	1.1	20	4.2	35	7.4	50	10.5
6	1.3	21	4.4	36	7.6	51	10.7
7	1.5	22	4.6	37	7.8	52	10.9
8	1.7	23	4.8	38	8.0	53	11.1
9	1.9	24	5.0	39	8.2	54	11.3
10	2.1	25	5.3	40	8.4	55	11.6
11	2.3	26	5.5	41	8.6	56	11.8
12	2.5	27	5.7	42	8.8	57	12.0
13	2.7	28	5.9	43	9.0	58	12.2
14	2.9	29	6.1	44	9.2	59	12.4
15	3.2	30	6.3	45	9.5	60	12.6

THE CONNORS COUNT™ CHART E

Time (minutes)	Points	Time (minutes)	Points	Time (minutes)	Points	Time (minutes)	Points
1	0.2	16	3.8	31	7.4	46	11.0
2	0.5	17	4.1	32	7.7	47	11.3
3	0.7	18	4.3	33	7.9	48	11.5
4	1.0	19	4.6	34	8.2	49	11.8
5	1.2	20	4.8	35	8.4	50	12.0
6	1.4	21	5.0	36	8.6	51	12.2
7	1.7	22	5.3	37	8.9	52	12.5
8	1.9	23	5.5	38	9.1	53	12.7
9	2.2	24	5.8	39	9.4	54	13.0
10	2.4	25	6.0	40	9.6	55	13.2
11	2.6	26	6.2	41	9.8	56	13.4
12	2.9	27	6.5	42	10.1	57	13.7
13	3.1	28	6.7	43	10.3	58	13.9
14	3.4	29	7.0	44	10.6	59	14.2
15	3.6	30	7.2	45	10.8	60	14.4

THE CONNORS COUNT® CHART F

Time (minutes)	Points	Time (minutes)	Points	Time (minutes)	Points	Time (minutes)	Points
1	0.3	16	4.8	31	9.3	46	13.8
2	0.6	17	5.1	32	9.6	47	14.1
3	0.9	18	5.4	33	9.9	48	14.4
4	1.2	19	5.7	34	10.2	49	14.7
5	1.5	20	6.0	35	10.5	50	15.0
6	1.8	21	6.3	36	10.8	51	15.3
7	2.1	22	6.6	37	11.1	52	15.6
8	2.4	23	6.9	38	11.4	53	15.9
9	2.7	24	7.2	39	11.7	54	16.2
10	3.0	25	7.5	40	12.0	55	16.5
11	3.3	26	7.8	41	12.3	56	16.8
12	3.6	27	8.1	42	12.6	57	17.1
13	3.9	28	8.4	43	12.9	58	17.4
14	4.2	29	8.7	44	13.2	59	17.7
15	4.5	30	9.0	45	13.5	60	18.0

THE CONNORS COUNT® CHART G

Time (minutes)	Points	Time (minutes)	Points	Time (minutes)	Points	Time (minutes)	Points
1	0.4	16	5.8	31	11.2	46	16.6
2	0.7	17	6.1	32	11.5	47	16.9
3	1.1	18	6.5	33	11.9	48	17.3
4	1.4	19	6.8	34	12.2	49	17.6
5	1.8	20	7.2	35	12.6	50	18.0
6	2.2	21	7.6	36	13.0	51	18.4
7	2.5	22	7.9	37	13.3	52	18.7
8	2.9	23	8.3	38	13.7	53	19.1
9	3.2	24	8.6	39	14.0	54	19.4
10	3.6	25	9.0	40	14.4	55	19.8
11	4.0	26	9.4	41	14.8	56	20.2
12	4.3	27	9.7	42	15.1	57	20.5
13	4.7	28	10.1	43	15.5	58	20.9
14	5.0	29	10.4	44	15.8	59	21.2
15	5.4	30	10.8	45	16.2	60	21.6

THE CONNORS COUNT™ CHART H

Time (minutes)	Points	Time (minutes)	Points	Time (minutes)	Points	Time (minutes)	Points
1	0.4	16	6.7	31	13.0	46	19.3
2	0.8	17	7.1	32	13.4	47	19.7
3	1.3	18	7.6	33	13.9	48	20.2
4	1.7	19	8.0	34	14.3	49	20.6
5	2.1	20	8.4	35	14.7	50	21.0
6	2.5	21	8.8	36	15.1	51	21.4
7	2.9	22	9.2	37	15.5	52	21.8
8	3.4	23	9.7	38	16.0	53	22.3
9	3.8	24	10.1	39	16.4	54	22.7
10	4.2	25	10.5	40	16.8	55	23.1
11	4.6	26	10.9	41	17.2	56	23.5
12	5.0	27	11.3	42	17.6	57	23.9
13	5.5	28	11.8	43	18.1	58	24.4
14	5.9	29	12.2	44	18.5	59	24.8
15	6.3	30	12.6	45	18.9	60	25.2

THE CONNORS COUNT® CHART I

Time (minutes)	Points	Time (minutes)	Points	Time (minutes)	Points	Time (minutes)	Points
1	0.5	16	7.7	31	14.9	46	22.1
2	1.0	17	8.2	32	15.4	47	22.6
3	1.4	18	8.6	33	15.8	48	23.0
4	1.9	19	9.1	34	16.3	49	23.5
5	2.4	20	9.6	35	16.8	50	24.0
6	2.9	21	10.1	36	17.3	51	24.5
7	3.4	22	10.6	37	17.8	52	25.0
8	3.8	23	11.0	38	18.2	53	25.4
9	4.3	24	11.5	39	18.7	54	25.9
10	4.8	25	12.0	40	19.2	55	26.4
11	5.3	26	12.5	41	19.7	56	26.9
12	5.8	27	13.0	42	20.2	57	27.4
13	6.2	28	13.4	43	20.6	58	27.8
14	6.7	29	13.9	44	21.1	59	28.3
15	7.2	30	14.4	45	21.6	60	28.8

THE CONNORS COUNT® CHART J

Time (minutes)	Points	Time (minutes)	Points	Time (minutes)	Points	Time (minutes)	Points
1	0.5	16	8.6	31	16.7	46	24.8
2	1.1	17	9.2	32	17.3	47	25.4
3	1.6	18	9.7	33	17.8	48	25.9
4	2.2	19	10.3	34	18.4	49	26.5
5	2.7	20	10.8	35	18.9	50	27.0
6	3.2	21	11.3	36	19.4	51	27.5
7	3.8	22	11.9	37	20.0	52	28.1
8	4.3	23	12.4	38	20.5	53	28.6
9	4.9	24	13.0	39	21.1	54	29.2
10	5.4	25	13.5	40	21.6	55	29.7
11	5.9	26	14.0	41	22.1	56	30.2
12	6.5	27	14.6	42	22.7	57	30.8
13	7.0	28	15.1	43	23.2	58	31.3
14	7.6	29	15.7	44	23.8	59	31.9
15	8.1	30	16.2	45	24.3	60	32.4

THE CONNORS COUNT® CHART K

Time (minutes)	Points	Time (minutes)	Points	Time (minutes)	Points	Time (minutes)	Points
1	0.6	16	9.6	31	18.6	46	27.6
2	1.2	17	10.2	32	19.2	47	28.2
3	1.8	18	10.8	33	19.8	48	28.8
4	2.4	19	11.4	34	20.4	49	29.4
5	3.0	20	12.0	35	21.0	50	30.0
6	3.6	21	12.6	36	21.6	51	30.6
7	4.2	22	13.2	37	22.2	52	31.2
8	4.8	23	13.8	38	22.8	53	31.8
9	5.4	24	14.4	39	23.4	54	32.4
10	6.0	25	15.0	40	24.0	55	33.0
11	6.6	26	15.6	41	24.6	56	33.6
12	7.2	27	16.2	42	25.2	57	34.2
13	7.8	28	16.8	43	25.8	58	34.8
14	8.4	29	17.4	44	26.4	59	35.4
15	9.0	30	18.0	45	27.0	60	36.0

THE CONNORS COUNT® CHART L

Time (minutes)	Points	Time (minutes)	Points	Time (minutes)	Points	Time (minutes)	Points
1	0.7	16	10.6	31	20.5	46	30.4
2	1.3	17	11.2	32	21.1	47	31.0
3	2.0	18	11.9	33	21.8	48	31.7
4	2.6	19	12.5	34	22.4	49	32.3
5	3.3	20	13.2	35	23.1	50	33.0
6	4.0	21	13.9	36	23.8	51	33.7
7	4.6	22	14.5	37	24.4	52	34.3
8	5.3	23	15.2	38	25.1	53	35.0
9	5.9	24	15.8	39	25.7	54	35.6
10	6.6	25	16.5	40	26.4	55	36.3
11	7.3	26	17.2	41	27.1	56	37.0
12	7.9	27	17.8	42	27.7	57	37.6
13	8.6	28	18.5	43	28.4	58	38.3
14	9.2	29	19.1	44	29.0	59	38.9
15	9.9	30	19.8	45	29.7	60	39.6

THE CONNORS COUNT® CHART M

Time (minutes)	Points	Time (minutes)	Points	Time (minutes)	Points	Time (minutes)	Points
1	0.7	16	11.5	31	22.3	46	33.1
2	1.4	17	12.2	32	23.0	47	33.8
3	2.2	18	13.0	33	23.8	48	34.6
4	2.9	19	13.7	34	24.5	49	35.3
5	3.6	20	14.4	35	25.2	50	36.0
6	4.3	21	15.1	36	25.9	51	36.7
7	5.0	22	15.8	37	26.6	52	37.4
8	5.8	23	16.6	38	27.4	53	38.2
9	6.5	24	17.3	39	28.1	54	38.9
10	7.2	25	18.0	40	28.8	55	39.6
11	7.9	26	18.7	41	29.5	56	40.3
12	8.6	27	19.4	42	30.2	57	41.0
13	9.4	28	20.2	43	31.0	58	41.8
14	10.1	29	20.9	44	31.7	59	42.5
15	10.8	30	21.6	45	32.4	60	43.2

THE CONNORS COUNT® CHART N

Time (minutes)	Points	Time (minutes)	Points	Time (minutes)	Points	Time (minutes)	Points
1	0.8	16	12.5	31	24.2	46	35.9
2	1.6	17	13.3	32	25.0	47	36.7
3	2.3	18	14.0	33	25.7	48	37.4
4	3.1	19	14.8	34	26.5	49	38.2
5	3.9	20	15.6	35	27.3	50	39.0
6	4.7	21	16.4	36	28.1	51	39.8
7	5.5	22	17.2	37	28.9	52	40.6
8	6.2	23	17.9	38	29.6	53	41.3
9	7.0	24	18.7	39	30.4	54	42.1
10	7.8	25	19.5	40	31.2	55	42.9
11	8.6	26	20.3	41	32.0	56	43.7
12	9.4	27	21.1	42	32.8	57	44.5
13	10.1	28	21.8	43	33.5	58	45.2
14	10.9	29	22.6	44	34.3	59	46.0
15	11.7	30	23.4	45	35.1	60	46.8

Exercising Your Options: Recommended Aerobic Activities

OPTIONS 1: • walking • stationary cycling (legs only or dual-action) • bicycling • cross-country skiing (with simulator) • swimming • rowing (with simulator) • tennis and other similar sports, provided running and jumping are kept to a minimum • low-impact aerobic dance

OPTIONS 2: • fast walking • jogging* • jumping rope* • stair climbing/stepping* • stationary cycling (legs only or dual-action) • cross-country skiing (outdoors or with simulator) • aerobic dance* • walking up an incline* • bicycling • rowing (outdoors or with simulator) • tennis, basketball, volleyball, and other similar ball games* • swimming

In my 16-week programs, I ask you to walk, jog, stationary cycle (dual-action), or jump rope for the aerobic portion of your workouts. Of course, you are free to use any of a variety of other aerobic exercises. To help you in deciding which are suitable alternatives I have divided your major options (there are many more) into two groups. Option 1 activities are those aerobic exercises than can be performed at a low or moderate intensity and do not place much impact or stress on your muscles, bones, or joints. These activities are suitable even for sedentary adults and can be performed with a low risk of injury. Option 2 activities are those aerobic exercises that are particularly suitable for working out at moderate or higher intensity. Some do place significant impact forces or stress on your musculoskeletal system and are therefore associated with a higher risk of injury—they are identified by means of an asterisk and are best avoided by people with orthopedic problems involving their weight-bearing joints and those of you who are considerably overweight. Certain activities are included in both option categories, which means that they are suitable for low as well as higher intensity exercise and do not place you at a significant risk for injury.

Using the Connors Count to Assess the Effectiveness of Your Weekly Workouts

Your goal is to earn between 35 and 100 points on the Connors Count each week during exercise. Exceeding 100 points does not provide substantially more benefit and is unnecessary from a health-related fitness standpoint. To gain optimal benefit, you should earn your weekly quota of points during the course of at least three workouts spread evenly throughout the week.

CONNORS COUNT	INTERPRETATION
Less than 25 points per week	**A start.** You're on your way.
25–34 points per week	**Better.** Come on, you can do it.
35–49 points per week	**Good.** Congratulations, you've counted yourself in.
50–74 points per week	**Very Good.** Keep it up—you're doing well.
75–99 points per week	**Excellent.** Be proud of yourself.
100 points per week	**Outstanding.** Unless you're planning to turn pro, you don't need any more points than this.

8

Eliminating the F Word

ALL RIGHT, I'll admit it. In my day, I've been known to let loose with an F word or two. Well, I'm working on that. I really am. But there is one F word I never say, and that's "failure." This word is not in my vocabulary and I want to encourage you to eliminate it from yours. Forever.

We all screw up once in a while. We're probably supposed to. It's one of the unwritten laws of life. But screwing up is not the same as failing. Not even close. The only way to fail, according to Connors' Law, is by not trying. When you don't try, you're being a nonparticipant. It's not that you have to try everything—you don't. But you shouldn't sit on the sidelines because you're afraid of failing. That's what failure is—sitting on the sidelines of life.

If you have ever started a fitness program and then dropped it, you are not alone. Millions of people have done the same thing. The trick is to isolate the reasons why the program did not work for you and try to avoid them the next time. Was it too difficult? Start slowly this time, and work up gradually. Was it not challenging enough? The Jimmy Connors Program B is plenty challenging. Too time-consuming? Once you've figured out the amount of points you can earn on the Connors Count in a given day *before* you begin my program, you may not need to spend nearly the time working out that you thought you did. Were you injured? Neil has included safety guidelines for you in Chapter 6 which minimize your risk of injury. Did you get bored or lose interest? Find some new activities that are more enjoyable to you and work out with friends and/or family members for moral support. Was it often a struggle to get to the gym? My program can be done anywhere—at the gym, at home, or on the road. Did the dog chew up your running shoes? Buy a better pair for yourself to celebrate your starting this new program (and while you're at it, pick up a bone for your dog).

Any of these might have seemed to be valid reasons for not continuing to exercise, at the time. But take it from me, when the weeks, months, and years go by and you can no longer fit into the clothes you want to wear, you don't have the stamina to walk around the block, or, God forbid, you should have a heart attack, I guarantee that none of those reasons will make you feel better.

Now that you've seen my program, I think you'll agree I've eliminated many of the potential problems associated with a regular workout routine. Once you get into the program of your choice, I believe you'll want to continue with it for a lifetime.

This doesn't mean you'll wake up every morning feeling like you can't wait to work out. I don't. There are days when I'm just not in the mood. Fortunately, you don't always have to be in the mood to exercise. You don't get extra points for doing the exercises with a smile on your face, but sometimes you just have to do it anyway. For me, those are the times when I feel the best about my workout—when I was tempted to skip it but resisted the temptation and put out the effort instead.

Of course, there *are* days when I do skip it. Nobody has to exercise seven days a week. As I told you in Chapter 4, that isn't necessarily better than exercising three to five days out of the week. In fact, it could make you more prone to injury. Rather than decide on that day whether or not I'm going to work out, I like to plan my nonexercise days in advance. Of course, this is purely a matter of choice, but it gives me a psychological edge to know that *I* decided to take the day off and it wasn't because I succumbed to the temptation to blow off the responsibility.

Still, there are times when things just come up and you can't stick to a schedule no matter how good your intentions. Don't feel bad if you miss a workout or two. Expect that things are going to happen that are beyond our control. It's called life. And life wouldn't be nearly as much fun if we knew everything in advance. Missing a few opportunities doesn't mean you've failed. Please don't think you have to give up on another fitness program just because you got busy at work, went on a business trip, took a vacation, had live-in guests, caught a cold, or sprained your ankle. Don't forget, my program is designed to work with your life—not to make you feel guilty for living it.

Rather than viewing a brief relapse back to inactivity as a failure, treat it as a challenge and try to get back on track as soon as possible. There are even ways to protect yourself when you're not following your normal schedule. When on a trip, pack your athletic shoes and a jump rope. If your hotel doesn't have a gym, you can work out in the room. I *never* leave home without my rope and I almost always find an occasion to use it. Sometimes I'll get up early when I'm on the road and run quietly up and down the hallways or around the block. If the family is with me, we make it a point to walk around the city and see the sights. You can put the Connors Count to use anytime, anywhere, with just a bit of planning and a dose of creativity.

Try to keep in mind that some of the health benefits of regular exercise are lost after as little as 2 or 3 days of abstinence. When it comes to your fitness level, you can expect a rapid deterioration during the first 2 or 3 weeks of not exercising. But, and I think this is great news, while completely stopping exercise produces a dramatic setback in your cardiorespiratory fitness level and strength, reducing the amount of exercise produces little or no setback for up to 15 weeks, if done correctly.

Remember the FIT concept (frequency, intensity, and time)? You can cut back the time allotted for your workout sessions and the frequency at which you do them by as much as two-thirds, but as long you keep the intensity at the same level, your cardiorespiratory fitness will remain unchanged for as long as 15 weeks. For example, if you usually walk briskly for 45 minutes at an intensity of a 13 on the Borg Scale, you can walk at the same pace (or faster) but reduce the time to 15 minutes. The same applies to strength training. You can cut back your sessions from two or three days a week to one day a week without experiencing a loss in strength as long as you lift the same amount of weight or keep the same degree of resistance.

What does this mean to you? During those times when you are unable to stick to your usual program, to maintain the health-promotion and functional-fitness benefits of your exercise program you should do the following:

1. Perform aerobic exercise at least every third day.
2. Perform the aerobic exercise at your usual intensity or RPE but reduce the duration by as much as two-thirds.
3. If possible, try to get in your usual strength training workout at least once a week.

If you follow these guidelines, not only will you maintain your benefit but if you can keep the period of reduced training to under 3 weeks, you may find yourself feeling refreshed and more fit than ever when you return to your usual workout routine. I know I do. This is why I always cut back on my training right before a major tournament. It allows me to enter the tournament relaxed and rejuvenated. I do the same thing whenever the family takes a vacation.

Naturally, if you are in the first few weeks of my program and cut back dramatically, you won't have many benefits to maintain. That's why I recommend your staying with the program for the full 16 weeks before deviating. But even that is sometimes impossible. When this happens, I won't count you out and I don't want you to count yourself out either. The Jimmy Connors program welcomes you back whenever you're ready. To ensure your safety, however, I will suggest that if you completely stop exercising for a week and want to begin the program again, return to the beginning of the last week of the program that you fully completed before you stopped. If you miss two weeks, go back to the start of the next-to-last week you fully completed before you stopped. Let's say, you were in Week 8 of my program and stopped exercising for two weeks. When you start working out again, you'd begin in Week 6. The formula is the same for all breaks in its continuity; you simply go back a week for every seven-day period you missed.

Once you make it through the 16-week mark, you'll be feeling and looking so good that the thought of missing a week of exercise will be a distressing one. I'd be willing to bet that after 16 weeks with the Jimmy Connors Workout, you will never want to go back to a life without regular exercise again. Now, how's that for a challenge?

To help you keep track of your progress, I recommend that you record your daily efforts in a training diary, at least for the first month or two. Once you're hooked, a training diary may not be necessary. But in the beginning of any new program, it is inspirational to be able to see in writing just how far you've come. I kept a training diary after my wrist injury and found it to be a big help.

To make things easy for you, I've included a sample of an empty training diary page. You might want to make a bunch of photocopies and stick them in a loose-leaf binder. On each page there is a place to record the type of activity you did (it doesn't matter whether the activity was a formal exercise or part of your daily routine), the number of minutes you did it, the rating of perceived exertion on the Borg Scale, and the number of points you earned on the Connors Count.

At the end of each week, there is a place to rate your enjoyment level and overall degree of satisfaction with the program. If you rate your score below a 3 for more than two consecutive weeks, you need to change your workout routine in one of the many possible ways we've already discussed.

You'll also notice that I have left a space on the training diary page for you to write in comments about your workouts. The purpose of this is to get you to be aware of how your workouts make you feel. The Borg Scale and the Connors Count are intended not only to ensure that you do enough exercise but also to prevent you from doing too much.

I know that there are some of you who still think if

a little is good then a lot must be better. Well, sometimes a lot isn't good at all. Not if you get hurt or sick or burned out. When this happens, you'll have to stop the program and may feel as if you've failed. I'm not about to let that happen to you. I've asked Neil to put together a list of indicators that could serve as a warning that you're doing too much. Listen to your body and be aware of the possible signs of overtraining. Keep in mind that some illnesses may cause similar symptoms. If you're in doubt, consult your doctor. If you are experiencing any of the following and you know it's because you're overdoing it, cut back on the frequency, intensity, and/or time of your workouts— even if they came from my program:

- Impaired physical performance—especially an inability to complete routine workouts that were no special challenge before, or higher than usual RPE scores during your workouts.
- Loss of weight without dieting or increasing exercise.
- For those of you who monitor your heart rate, a higher than usual increase in your heart rate during workouts.
- A heavy or sluggish feeling in your legs when working out.
- Dizziness when you stand up.
- Tiredness or listlessness that lasts longer than 24 hours after workouts.
- Muscle and joint pains.
- Muscle soreness that is persistent and worsens from workout to workout.

- Swelling of lymph glands.
- Diarrhea and other gastrointestinal disturbances.
- Greater susceptibility to allergies and headaches.
- Greater susceptibility to injuries.
- Longer healing periods for minor cuts and scratches.
- In premenopausal women, irregular or no monthly menstruation.
- General loss of motivation, drive, or enthusiasm for life.
- Inability to think about anything else but your next workout.
- Workouts become unenjoyable.
- Feeling of depression and/or anxiety.
- Easy irritation.
- Insomnia or other changes in sleep patterns.
- Loss of appetite.
- Loss of libido or interest in sex.
- Poor coordination and general clumsiness.

Again, any one of these signs can mean something other than that you're overtraining. But to keep you healthy and happy with the program, I wanted to make you aware of them so you'd be safe now instead of sorry later.

THE JIMMY CONNORS WORKOUT PROGRAM
TRAINING DIARY

Monday (date ———)	Tuesday (date ———)	Wednesday (date ———)

Activity:
Time:
RPE:
  Points =
	Activity:
	Time:
	RPE:
	  Points =
		Activity:
		Time:
		RPE:
		  Points =

Activity:
Time:
RPE:
  Points =
	Activity:
	Time:
	RPE:
	  Points =
		Activity:
		Time:
		RPE:
		  Points =

Activity:
Time:
RPE:
  Points =
	Activity:
	Time:
	RPE:
	  Points =
		Activity:
		Time:
		RPE:
		  Points =

Activity:
Time:
RPE:
  Points =
	Activity:
	Time:
	RPE:
	  Points =
		Activity:
		Time:
		RPE:
		  Points =

Activity:
Time:
RPE:
  Points =
	Activity:
	Time:
	RPE:
	  Points =
		Activity:
		Time:
		RPE:
		  Points =

Activity:
Time:
RPE:
  Points =
Connors Count
=
	Activity:
	Time:
	RPE:
	  Points =
	Connors Count
	=
		Activity:
		Time:
		RPE:
		  Points =
		Connors Count
		=

COMMENTS

Thursday (date ———)	Friday (date ———)	Saturday (date ———)	Sunday (date ———)
Activity:	Activity:	Activity:	Activity:
Time:	Time:	Time:	Time:
RPE:	RPE:	RPE:	RPE:
Points =	Points =	Points =	Points =
Activity:	Activity:	Activity:	Activity:
Time:	Time:	Time:	Time:
RPE:	RPE:	RPE:	RPE:
Points =	Points =	Points =	Points =
Activity:	Activity:	Activity:	Activity:
Time:	Time:	Time:	Time:
RPE:	RPE:	RPE:	RPE:
Points =	Points =	Points =	Points =
Activity:	Activity:	Activity:	Activity:
Time:	Time:	Time:	Time:
RPE:	RPE:	RPE:	RPE:
Points =	Points =	Points =	Points =
Activity:	Activity:	Activity:	Activity:
Time:	Time:	Time:	Time:
RPE:	RPE:	RPE:	RPE:
Points =	Points =	Points =	Points =
Activity:	Activity:	Activity:	Activity:
Time:	Time:	Time:	Time:
RPE:	RPE:	RPE:	RPE:
Points =	Points =	Points =	Points =
Connors Count =	Connors Count =	Connors Count =	Connors Count =

ENJOYMENT RATING FOR WEEK (circle number):

1. Very unenjoyable
2. Unenjoyable
3. Somewhat enjoyable
4. Enjoyable
5. Very enjoyable

CONNORS COUNT TOTAL FOR WEEK =

Beyond Exercise

BY NOW YOU SHOULD fully understand how important doing the right amount of exercise is in relation to
both the quality and the length of your life. The Connors Count will ensure that you have the information
you need to do just that. You should also realize that
you probably don't need as much exercise as you
thought you did to receive great benefits and that a
regular exercise program doesn't have to intrude on
your lifestyle. It can and *should* complement all the
other facets of your daily routine. This brings me to the
last point I want to make in my book, one that I feel
very strongly about. There is more to health and fitness
than just working out.

By reading this book and following either of these

programs, you've taken a giant step toward bettering your life. But I don't want you to think that exercise is the entire answer, because it isn't. I would rather you consider exercise as one very important part of a healthy lifestyle. To get the most results from a *health-promotion* standpoint, the Jimmy Connors Workout Program should be combined with many other positive lifestyle factors that you've heard before but should be mentioned here: not smoking, eating correctly, learning to cope with stress, staying as far away from drugs as you can, alcohol in moderation only, practicing safe sex, wearing seatbelts in the car, and getting regular medical check-ups.

We all need to go *beyond exercise* to receive the gifts a healthy lifestyle has to offer and to stay a participant for as long as possible. I mean, what's the point of putting out the effort of exercising regularly and bothering to keep track of our Connors Count℠ score only to risk our lives somewhere else? This is something that I have recently taken very much to heart. I had a tendency to drive much too fast, just for the thrill of it. I thought it was fun to test myself on how quickly I could get from point A to point B. And I don't know if it has had something to do with turning 40 or not, but I have gotten wiser. My life is getting more enjoyable every day and no *cheap thrill* is worth destroying what I've worked so hard to achieve.

It is also very important that you understand that the concept of fitness isn't limited to how far you can run, how much weight you can lift, or how flexible you are. It's much more than that. It is having the ability to balance all the elements in your life. I want to be as fit mentally, emotionally, and spiritually as I am physically.

You already know what I mean by *physical fitness.* I shared my programs with you because they work. I think my success not only as a professional tennis player but as a *40-year-old* professional tennis player has proved that. My programs aren't a cram session in physical fitness, but a way of life. I want to touch briefly on the other three elements of *total fitness* and tell you a little about what they mean to me and how they can benefit you.

Mental fitness is about exercising your mind. It involves being aware of what's happening in your neighborhood, your city, your state, your country, and the world. There are many ways of giving your mind a workout. I like reading the paper—not just the sports section, but all of it—cover to cover. Books are another great source of information for me. They can take me to places I've only thought about (or only have seen from a hotel room and tennis court) and make me feel as though I've been there. I want to be articulate, to be able to participate in any number of conversations on a variety of subjects.

If I were capable of talking only about tennis or what I do for a workout, I'd be a pretty dull person. I don't want that. It's exhilarating for me to learn about what makes other people tick. I'm interested. Even if I don't agree with an opinion, it's good for me to listen and at least try to understand the reasoning behind it. I don't think I've ever met a person who couldn't teach me something.

My mother encouraged this kind of curiosity in me as a small child. She saw to it that my life consisted of other things besides tennis. There was time set aside every day for homework and for playing with my friends. She didn't want me to be one-dimensional or to grow up believing that tennis was my only option.

As you know, my mom was (and still is) my coach. But it was *my* decision to become the best in the world. I told her that was my goal when I was 10 years old. I remember laying it on her one day on the way home from practice. She pulled the car over to the side of the road and looked into my eyes to see if I meant it. I did. Even then, she would not allow me to give up everything else. We had a goal to work toward, but my mom is a smart lady. She knew that if I made tennis my whole life, I'd get burnt out quickly. Instinctively, she knew that in order for me to get to the top and stay at the top, tennis would always have to be fun. And it has been. But only because I had other diversions.

What I'm trying to say is that there is life after exercise. Please don't become so obsessed with working out that you lose sight of what you're supposed to work out *for*. That kind of obsession can't last forever. You'll either get sick, get hurt, or give up on the program.

Emotional fitness goes hand in hand with mental and physical fitness. You already know that physical activity is essential for keeping emotions in check. It allows us to blow off steam and clear our heads before saying or doing something we'll regret later. It also helps me to keep my mind on whatever I'm doing at the moment. This lesson was an important one for me, one I learned the hard way.

I had thought about getting married and having a family since I was 15 years old. Meeting and marrying my wife, Patti, was the best thing that ever happened to me. Having Brett and Aubree is a joy no words can adequately describe.

When I got married, I was at the height of my career. Patti knew and understood from the beginning what the sacrifices would be. That didn't make our lifestyle easy. We traveled from city to city, and country to country, in and out of hotels one after another. A crowd of people was always around us, making our time alone together very limited. And when we were at home I spent a lot of time practicing. Although I was trying to build a foundation for our future, I had to take into consideration what she must have been feeling. I wanted her to know how much it meant to me to have her there.

When Brett was born, I was thrilled to have them both with me on the road. Things were a little more hectic. Now, in addition to our luggage, the crowds, and my racquets, we lugged around strollers, playpens, and bottles. It was fun and I wouldn't have traded it for anything. Knowing they were watching gave me more to play for, more to win for.

Pretty soon, though, Brett had to start school and Patti wasn't about to leave him alone. Although I was never actually alone on the road, I was often lonely without the family. I didn't want to miss anything. Then Aubree was born and I thought, "Hey, what am I doing? I've wanted this for as long as I can remember, and I'm not around to enjoy it." But I couldn't just quit. Now I had even more reason to keep playing. You see, when I first started in tennis, the money wasn't anything like it is today. Back then, you had to play *a lot* of matches in order to make a comfortable living. For a while I had contemplated going to law school, but gave it up when I realized I could make a career out of doing what I do best. I didn't really have another choice at that moment. I had two children to raise and for whom to provide an education. Besides, I loved the game. But I was trying to be two places at once and it was killing me.

When I was on the road, I worried about Patti and the kids. Were they safe? How was Brett doing in school? Would I be away when Aubree took her first steps? When I was at home with them, I felt I should be working at tennis. I knew the more I practiced, the more I'd win. The more I'd win, the better their future would be. It was like being on an emotional roller coaster.

I knew I had to make a change, and I did. It wasn't the kind of change that anyone outside the circle of my family and closest friends would have noticed, but it was significant. What I did was sort of discipline my emotions. I taught myself to concentrate on what I was doing at the time. When I was practicing, I practiced hard. I tried not to think about anything but the game when I was on the court, whether at home or on the road. But when I was with the family, I was with them 100 percent. They had my undivided attention. This has worked for me ever since. Now I have my family and friends, a business to run, and tennis. I've found the time for all of it.

If you are having trouble keeping your emotions in

check, look at yourself the way I did. It may help. It is possible that you're trying to be in too many places at the same time. When that happens, everything suffers. Hey, we're only human. We are entitled to feel every emotion, we just have to make them work to our benefit. There is no crime in taking time off from the job to relax and enjoy the things we work *for*. But if you're thinking about playing the whole time you're working and about working the whole time you're playing, you don't get much from either. If you can learn the value of keeping your mind on what's in front of you, you'll get the most both worlds have to offer.

I know many people who say they feel guilty about coming home to the family after a long day and heading straight for a workout, just like I used to feel. The best advice I can give you is to try to involve your family in exercise and make it something you can all do together. If that's not possible, sit down and talk to them about why exercise is so important—that it will keep you with them longer. If you can make them understand, they'll be upset if you *don't* work out. You see, exercise should be important not only to you but to all those you love and care about.

The last component in a balanced fitness plan is *spiritual fitness*. I'm not talking about religion, although religion can certainly be included in this element. What I mean is being satisfied with the kind of person you are on the *inside*. Nothing I've earned or done would mean anything to me if I didn't feel I had gotten it with integrity. I'm no preacher and I've never been mistaken for a saint, but I do have a code of ethics by which I live.

I'm not just Jimmy Connors the tennis pro anymore. I'm one-half of Mr. and Mrs. Connors and one-fourth of the Connors family. My kids are depending on me to show them the way. *I'm* depending on me to show them the *right* way. Again, I owe this to my mom. She said a long time ago, "Jimbo, when you're on the court you can be a tiger. You fight for what you want and be proud of your efforts. Off the court, you're just like anyone else. You must respect women, set an example for your children, and earn your friendships. The only kind of man worth being is a gentleman." And she was right. I'm not only proud of the things I've accomplished, but *how* I've accomplished them. I know I'm a lucky man, and it seems that the harder I work, the luckier I get.

The same can be true for you. While I'll be the first to say that exercise isn't everything, it will make your life richer in many ways. It can't take the place of loving relationships, although it can make them more fulfilling. It can't pay the mortgage, yet it can give you the energy you need to work harder. Exercise itself won't bring you more friends, but by relieving stress, it can make you friendlier. What I'm trying to say is that exercise is a tool to be used and enjoyed in many ways and for many reasons.

So, my friends, there you have it. The Connors formula for balanced fitness. Take it and do with it what you please. I don't think you'll be disappointed if you can remember these three things: work hard, play often, and don't forget to look up every now and then to say, "Thanks."

Afterword: The Ball's in Your Court

I want you to know what a pleasure it has been for me to share my workout program. For many of you, it won't be the first program you've tried, but I believe it may be the last. Not because it has worked for Jimmy Connors the tennis pro, but because it has worked and is *still working* for Jimmy Connors the 40-year-old, the father, the husband, the friend, and the person.

Just like you, I have a lot of stuff on my plate and I want to do it all well. And, just like you, things don't always turn out the way I plan them. But my workout program gives me the energy and the patience I need to keep trying. This is the only program out there I know about that gives you credit for doing the activities you do every day—before you actually begin working out. This program respects the fact that you have other priorities at certain times and applauds you for it. It's the only program out there I know of that allows you to work out at your own self-determined level of exertion, yet still ensures that you get the right amount of exercise. The Connors Count and the Borg Scale put you in the driver's seat of your life.

I have referred to the workout throughout this book as "my program." But I've given you so many opportunities to adjust it to suit your needs that I hope you'll refer to it as "our program" from now on. That would make me feel good.

I also hope that you'll keep in touch and let me know how you're doing. Feel free to write or come down and visit with me after a match. I'd like to hear about how the program made positive changes in your life. After all, I've already shared with you the changes this program has made in my life. One of the best things to come out of this program for me is that it has kept me around long enough so that you still know who the hell I am. And I want to take this opportunity to thank you for coming out to see me all these years. It means more than you could possibly know.

But it's not over yet. Who knows what's still to come? Like I said before, I won't let them count me out. And now you've got what it takes not to count yourself out either.

Recommended Reading List

American College of Sports Medicine. Position stand. The recommended quantity of exercise for developing and maintaining cardiorespiratory and muscle fitness in healthy adults. *Medicine and Science in Sports and Exercise* 1990: 22:265–274.

Cooper, K.H. *Aerobics.* New York: Bantam Books, 1968.

Evans, W., Rosenberg, I.H. *Biomarkers: The 10 Determinants of Aging You Can Control.* New York: Simon and Schuster, 1991.

Fletcher, G.F.; Blair S.N.; Blumenthal, J., et al. American Heart Association position statement on exercise. Benefits and recommendations for physical activity programs for all Americans. *Circulation* 1992: 86:340–344.

Fletcher, G.F.; Froelicher, V.F.; Hartly, H., et al. Exercise standards. A statement for health professionals from the American Heart Association. *Circulation* 1990: 82:2286–2322.

Gordon, N.F. *Chronic Fatigue: Your Complete Exercise Guide.* Champaign, IL: Leisure Press, 1992.

Gordon, N.F., Gibbons, L.W., *The Cooper Clinic Cardiac Rehabilitation Program.* New York: Simon and Schuster, 1990.

Jette, M.; Sidney, K.; Blumchen, G. Metabolic equivalents (METS) in exercise testing, exercise prescription, and evaluation of functional capacity. *Clinical Cardiology* 1990: 13:-555–565.

Solis, K.M. *Ropics: The Next Jump Forward in Fitness.* Champaign, IL: Leisure Press, 1992.

Yanker, G., Burton, K. *Walking Medicine.* New York: McGraw-Hill, 1990.

Index

aerobic (cardiorespiratory) fitness,
15–16, 34, 35, 36, 51–52,
57–59, 220, 221
aerobic exercise, 50, 52–53
amount needed for fitness, 51–52
cycling, 73, 84–85
dancing, 86–87
jogging, *see* jogging
jumping rope, *see* jumping rope
stair climbing, 77, 84, 112
stretching and, 73–74
swimming, 85–86
walking, *see* walking
aerobic workouts, 51–69
calories burned in, 64–66
Connors Count in, 66–69; *see also*
Connors Count
cooling down after, 97
frequency of, 53–54, 221
intensity of, 56–64
length of, 53, 54–56, 59, 221, 224
perceived level of exertion in, 61;
see also Borg Scale of
Perceived Exertion
plateau and, 52, 68–69
warm-up period in, 73, 97
see also workout programs
Agassi, Andre, 24–25
aging, 36
air pollution, 104
American College of Sports
Medicine, 70, 73, 92
American Heart Association, 52, 67
anaerobic exercise, 15, 16, 52
arthritis, 93

bandages, elastic, 100
Becker, Boris, 22, 25
bicycling, *see* cycling
bleeding, 100
blood pressure, 27, 43–44, 93, 95,
97
body, listening to, 2, 7, 16, 48, 51,
61, 113
warning signs of overtraining,
224–25
body fatness, 38, 40–41
see also weight loss
body temperature, 101–3, 105
bone problems, 43, 95
Borg, Gunnar, 61
Borg Scale of Perceived Exertion,
51, 61–64, 67, 68, 71, 76, 221,
237
Connors Count used with, 67–68;
see also Connor Count
RPE in, 61–63, 66, 68, 71, 81, 82,
87, 109–10, 221, 223, 224
breathlessness, 96

calorie burning (energy
expenditure), 40, 41, 43, 52,
57, 59–60, 80, 82, 84
in aerobic workouts, 64–66
Connors Count and, 66, 67
during sleep, 40–41
cancer, 43
cardiac conditions, *see* heart
conditions
cardiorespiratory fitness, 15–16, 34,
35, 36, 51–52, 57–59, 220, 221

cardiorespiratory fitness *(cont.)*
  see also aerobic exercise; aerobic
    workouts
Chang, Michael, 17–18, 62
chest pain or discomfort, 93, 94,
    95–96
children, 78
cholesterol, 93
chronic illnesses, 61, 92–93
cigarettes, 93, 104
clothing, 102, 103
colds, 105
compression, for injury, 100
Connors, Aubree, 21–22, 23, 34,
    232, 233
Connors, Brett, 16, 20, 23–24, 34,
    79, 87, 232, 233
Connors, Gloria, 17, 231, 235
Connors, Jimmy:
  at French Open, 17–18, 19, 62
  at U.S. Open, 11, 20–25
  at Wimbledon, 18–19
  workout program of, *see* Jimmy
    Connors Workout
  wrist injury of, 11–17, 18, 20,
    100, 223
Connors, Patti, 16, 20, 23, 24, 34,
    232, 233
Connors Count, 7, 48, 87, 218, 220,
    228, 229, 237
  in aerobic workouts, 66–69
  assessing workout effectiveness
    with, 213
  charts for, 110, 196–209
  everyday activities and, 76, 78,
    79, 88, 111–12, 223
  how to calculate points in,
    109–13
  index for, 110, 192–95
Connors' Law, 217
cooldowns, 96, 97
Cooper, Ken, 34
coronary heart disease, 43–44, 93
  see also heart conditions
cross-training, 97
cycle stress test, 61

cycling, 84–85
  warm-up for, 73

dancing, aerobic, 86–87
diabetes, 27, 43, 93
diary, training, 223, 226–27
diets, plateaus in, 41–43
disability zone, 35–36
disease prevention, 27, 29, 31, 33,
    38, 43–44, 57, 69
diseases, chronic, 92–93
  heart rate and, 61
dizziness, 94, 96, 101, 224
doctors, 92–95, 224
downtime, 78–79
dumbbells, 71
dynamic resistance exercises, 70

elderly people, 38
elevation, for injury, 101
emotional fitness, 43, 44–45, 231–34
endorphins, 45
endurance, muscular strength and,
    34, 35, 50
  see also muscular strength
    workouts
energy expenditure, *see* calorie
    burning
everyday activities, 76–79
  Connors Count points for, 76, 78,
    79, 88, 111–12, 223
  see also lifestyle
exercise:
  aerobic, *see* aerobic exercise
  anaerobic, 15, 16, 52
  benefits of, 67–68, 220
  determining how much is
    necessary, 50–74
  energy expended during, *see*
    calorie burning
  goals and, 3–4
  ideal, characteristics of, 80–81
  importance of, 228, 235
  lifestyle and, *see* lifestyle
  loss of health benefits after
    abstinence from, 220

moderate, 45–46, 50, 59, 60
motivation and, 32–33
obsession with, 48, 231
reducing amount of, 220–22
resistance, 70
safe, *see* safe exercise
types of, 79, 80–88
see also fitness; workout
   programs

failure, 217–25
fainting, 94, 96
family, 218, 234
fat, body, 38, 40–41
   see also weight loss
fatigue, 36
feet, 98–99
fever, 105
first-aid program, RICE, 99–101
FIT (Frequency, Intensity, Time),
   53–56, 59–60, 68, 221, 224
   see also intensity of workouts
fitness, 26–31
   aerobic, 15–16, 34, 35, 36, 51–52,
      57–59, 220, 221
   anaerobic, 15
   body fatness and, 38, 40–41; *see*
      also weight loss
   definitions of, 26–27, 31, 229–30
   as disease prevention, 27, 29, 31,
      33, 38, 43–44, 57, 69
   emotional, 43, 44–45, 231–34
   flexibility, 34, 35, 50
   functional, 29–30, 33–38, 221
   as health promotion, 29–30,
      38–46, 48, 221, 229
   health-related, 27–30, 33, 49, 51
   improvements in level of, 51–52,
      67–68
   mental, 44–45, 230–31
   moderate exercise and, 45–46, 50,
      59, 60
   muscular strength and endurance,
      34, 35, 50
   performance-related, 27, 28, 30,
      33, 49, 52

psychological well-being and, 38,
   43, 44–45
reasons for maintaining, 26–27,
   30
reducing amount of exercise and,
   220–22
spiritual, 234
stopping exercise and, 220
total, 230–35
   see also exercise; workout
      programs
flexibility, 34, 35, 50
   exercises for, *see* stretching
      exercises
flu, 105
fluids, 102
French Open, 17–18, 19, 62
frequency of workouts, 53–54, 59,
   219, 221, 224
functional fitness, 29–30

garden, working in, 78
Garrick, Jim, 13, 14
Gordon, Neil, 5, 6, 30, 35, 40, 46,
   61, 82, 91–92, 113

healthy lifestyle, 229
heart attacks, 27, 43–44, 48
heart (cardiac) conditions, 43–44,
   46, 57, 93, 94, 95
   heart rate and, 61, 224
   sudden death from, 46
   warning signs of, 95–96
   see also cardiorespiratory fitness
heat stroke, 101
high blood pressure, 27, 43–44, 93,
   95
hill jogging, 81, 82
hot weather, 102–3
humidity, 102
hydrocarbons, 104
hyperthermia, 101–3, 105

ice, to treat injury, 100
illnesses:
   chronic, 61, 92–93

illnesses *(cont.)*
  fever and, 105
  overtraining and, 224
  see also disease prevention
inactivity, 36, 43–44, 57, 69
inflammation, 100
injuries, 48, 53, 59, 80, 82, 83, 84,
      98, 103, 113, 218, 219, 225
  orthopedic, 98–101
  RICE treatment for, 99–101
  stretching and, 73–74
  see also safe exercise
intensity of workouts, 53, 56–64,
      221, 224
  measuring of, 60–64; *see also*
      Connors Count
isometric resistance exercises, 70

Jimmy Connors Workout, 6–7, 33,
      107–13, 237–38
  beginning again after stopping,
      222
  Connors Count in, *see* Connors
      Count
  length of program, 113
  options in, 109, 211–12
  personalizing of, 80, 109, 238
  Program A, 108, 112, 113,
      115–47
  Program A 4-Week Optional
      Extension, 108, 113, 149–57
  Program B, 108, 113, 159–91,
      218
  safety and, *see* safe exercise
  stopping program, 222, 224
  training diary for, 223, 226–27
jogging, 81–82
  hill, 81, 82
  jumping rope compared with, 83
  orthopedic injuries and, 99
  warm-up for, 73
joint problems, 95
jumping rope, 16, 79, 82–83,
      220
  jogging compared with, 83
  orthopedic injuries and, 99

lifestyle, 30, 70, 75–88, 228–29
  healthy, 229
  sedentary, 27, 30, 36, 43–44, 57, 69
  suggestions for improving, 77–78
lung disease, 93

McEnroe, John, 13, 19, 21
McEnroe, Patrick, 21, 22, 23
medical guidelines, *see* safe exercise
medications, 53–54, 101
mental fitness, 45–46, 230–31
moderate exercise, 50, 59, 60
moral support, 218
motivation, 32–33, 225
mowing the lawn, 78
muscles, 80
  calorie burning and, 40–41, 80
  soreness in, 224
muscular strength and endurance,
      34, 35, 50
muscular strength workouts, 69–73,
      221
  Borg Scale and, 71
  breathing and, 106
  using correct technique in, 105–6
  scheduling of, 71
  stopping exercise and, 220
  warm-up for, 73
myocarditis, 105

nausea, 96, 101
nitrogen dioxide, 104
Nuprin, 53–54

options, for Jimmy Connors
      Workout, 109, 211–12
orthopedic injuries, 98–101
osteoporosis, 43
overtraining, warning signs of,
      224–25
ozone, 104

pain and discomfort, 56, 95–96,
      100, 224
  in chest, 93, 94, 95–96
  stretching and, 74

perceived level of exertion, *see* Borg Scale of Perceived Exertion
Physical Activity Readiness Questionnaire (PAR-Q), 93, 94–95
physicians, 92–95, 224
points, *see* Connors Count
pollution, 104
pregnancy, 95
psychological well-being, 38, 43, 44–45
pulse:
  irregular, 96
  taking of, 61

rating of perceived exertion (RPE), 61–63, 66, 68, 71, 81, 82, 87, 109–10, 221, 223, 224
  see also Borg Scale of Perceived Exertion
recreational sports, 87
relaxation, 79
resistance exercises, 70
  see also muscular strength workouts
resting and reducing of exercise, after injury, 99–100
RICE treatment, 99–101
risks, 46–49
  see also disease prevention; heart conditions; injuries; safe exercise
rope jumping, *see* jumping rope
Rostagno, Derrick, 18–19
RPE, *see* rating of perceived exertion
running, *see* jogging

safe exercise, 91–106, 218
  cool down and, 96, 97
  doctor's supervision and, 92–95
  fever-associated illnesses and, 105
  frequency and, 106
  muscle-strengthening exercises and, 105–6

orthopedic injury prevention, 98–101
Physical Activity Readiness Questionnaire and, 93, 94–95
pollution and, 104
starting slowly and progressing gradually, 97–98
stopping workout program and, 222
warm-up and, 73, 74, 97
warning signs of impending cardiac complication, 95–96
weather conditions and, 101–3
  see also injuries
Scheinberg, Rick, 13, 14, 15
sedentary lifestyle, 27, 30, 36, 43–44, 57, 69
sedentary women, study of, 56–57
self-control, self-discipline vs., 30–31, 44
shoes, 98–99, 220
shortness of breath, 96
sleep, burning calories during, 40–41
smoking, 93, 104
spiritual fitness, 234
sprinting, 16
stair climbing, 77, 84, 112
standing in line, 78–79
stationary cycling, 84–85
strength and endurance, muscular, 34, 35, 50
  see also muscular strength workouts
stress, 45, 235
stress test, 61
stretching exercises, 50, 69, 73–74, 109
  aerobic exercise and, 73–74
  injury and, 73–74
stroke, 43, 93
sulfur dioxide, 104
sweating, 101, 102, 103
  fever and, 105
swelling, 100, 101
swimming, 85–86

team sports, 87
temperature, body, 101–3, 105
time (duration of exercise), 53,
    54–56, 59, 221, 224
time, lack of, 75–77, 218
total suspended particulates, 104
traffic, 85, 104
training diary, 223, 226–27
treadmills, 61, 82

U.S. Open, 11, 20–25

vacations, 220, 222
viral myocarditis, 105

waiting, 78–79
walking, 57, 77, 81–82, 112, 220,
    221
  with hand weights, 82
  to work, 77
walking the dog, 76–77
warming up, 73, 74, 97
warning signs:
  of impending cardiac
    complication, 95–96
  of overtraining, 224–25
water, 102
weather, 82, 84, 101–3
weight, body, energy expenditure
    and, 67
weight loss, 40–43, 102, 224
  see also calorie burning
weights, hand, walking with, 82

weight training, 50, 70–73
  see also muscular strength workouts
Wimbledon, 18–19
workout programs:
  aerobic exercise in, *see* aerobic
    workouts
  balanced, 34, 35, 50
  using Connors Count to assess
    effectiveness of, 213
  disability zone avoided with, 35–36
  dropping out of, 30–31, 218–20,
    224
  family and, 218, 234
  fitting into lifestyle, *see* lifestyle
  for flexibility, 34, 35, 50; *see also*
    stretching exercises
  frequency in, 53–54, 59, 219, 221,
    224
  gradual progress in, 68, 97–98, 218
  motivation for starting, 32–33
  for muscular strength, *see*
    muscular strength workouts
  potential problems in, 218–20
  psychological well-being fostered
    by, 38, 43, 44–45
  risks and, *see* risks
  safety in, *see* safe exercise
  starting of, at advanced age, 38
  three types of fitness targeted in,
    33–35, 50
  weight loss and, *see* weight loss
  see also exercise; fitness; Jimmy
    Connors Workout